Introducing Pharmacology
for Nursing and Healthcare

PEARSON

NURSING&HEALTH

FIRST FOR HEALTH

We work with leading authors to develop the strongest educational materials in nursing and healthcare, bringing cutting-edge thinking and best learning practice to a global market.

Under a range of well-known imprints, including Pearson Education, we craft high quality print and electronic publications that help readers to understand and apply their content, whether studying or at work.

To find out more about the complete range of our publishing, please visit us on the World Wide Web at: **www.pearsoned.co.uk**

Introducing Pharmacology
for Nursing and Healthcare

Roger McFadden

Harlow, England • London • New York • Boston • San Francisco • Toronto
Sydney • Tokyo • Singapore • Hong Kong • Seoul • Taipei • New Delhi
Cape Town • Madrid • Mexico City • Amsterdam • Munich • Paris • Milan

Pearson Education Limited
Edinburgh Gate
Harlow
Essex CM20 2JE
England

and Associated Companies throughout the world

Visit us on the World Wide Web at:
www.pearsoned.co.uk

First published 2009

ISBN: 978-0-273-71863-5

British Library Cataloguing-in-Publication Data
A catalogue record for this book is available from the British Library

Library of Congress Cataloging-in-Publication Data
McFadden, Roger.
 Introducing pharmacology for nursing and healthcare / Roger McFadden.
  p. ; cm.
 Includes bibliographical references and index.
 ISBN 978-0-273-71863-5
 1. Pharmacology. 2. Nursing. I. Title.
 [DNLM: 1. Pharmacology - Nurses' Instruction. 2. Drug Therapy - Nurses' Instruction.
 3. Pharmaceutical Preparations - Nurses' Instruction. QV 4 M4768i 2009]
 RM300.M34 2009
 615′.1—dc22

                                        2009014434

10 9 8 7 6 5 4 3 2 1
12 11 10 09

Typeset in 9.5/13pt Interstate Light by 35
Printed in Great Britain by Henry Ling Ltd, at the Dorset Press, Dorchester, Dorset

The publisher's policy is to use paper manufactured from sustainable forests.

Brief contents

Contents

Introduction

Welcome, reader, to the fascinating world of pharmacology.

You are probably reading this book because you have enrolled on a course of studies leading to a recognised clinical qualification such as Registered Nurse (RN) or Registered Midwife (RM). Alternatively, you may already be a registered practitioner but are returning to study in order to gain additional qualifications such as Nurse Independent Prescriber or Specialist Practitioner. Whatever your reason for studying the subject, you will find an understanding of pharmacology to be invaluable in your clinical practice. Therapeutic drugs are widely prescribed to patients in most branches of medicine and it is unlikely that any clinical practitioner will be working in an area where patients have not been prescribed some form of medication.

If you will be looking after patients who have been prescribed drugs, you need to understand the mechanism whereby those drugs work. For the patient, it will be sufficient to know that an analgesic drug relieves pain or an anxiolytic drug relieves anxiety but you, as a clinical practitioner, need to understand the action of the drugs at a much deeper level. You may have had the responsibility for the administration of a drug to a patient or perhaps you are looking after a patient who has been administered a drug by a clinical colleague. In either case, it is you who will be responsible for monitoring the patient's response to the drug, and not only must you ensure that the drug is working but also (and equally importantly) whether the drug is causing any unwanted side-effects. To do this effectively it is essential that you understand the drug's mechanism of action – how it produces its therapeutic effect. Increasingly, many non-medical practitioners, nurses, midwives, etc., are trained and licensed to prescribe independently, and a good understanding of pharmacology is absolutely essential.

The main problem associated with the study of pharmacology is that the subject makes little sense unless you also understand the related **anatomy, physiology** and **pathology** (disease). Let us explain further . . .

Pharmacology is the study of how drugs work in the human body and anyone who has ever opened a physiology textbook will know that the structure (anatomy) of the human body is rather complex and its workings (physiology) are even more complicated. Unfortunately, this means that the action of drugs on the body is equally complicated. Put simply, you cannot understand the pharmacology unless you first understand the anatomy and physiology. Visit your university or college library and you will find plenty of anatomy and physiology books, but most of them are fairly weighty and not particularly oriented to the study of pharmacology. Look on the adjacent shelves and you will find that there is no shortage of pharmacology books in the library. These will undoubtedly tell you all you need to know about pharmacology but they nearly all begin with the assumption that the reader arrives at the subject with a good understanding of basic anatomy and physiology. Experience has shown that this is not always the case and even when students have some background in human anatomy and physiology they can struggle with the specialised cell biology and biochemistry that underpins the subject of pharmacology.

So, in order to understand pharmacology, you need to understand basic anatomy and physiology and you also need to understand pathologies.

Apart from a few exceptions such as oral contraceptives, drugs are not prescribed to healthy people; mostly they have some disease or are at risk of developing a disease or complication. This means that most drugs can only be understood in the context of pathologies as that is where they have their prime source of action. For example, common analgesics such as *ibuprofen* and *diclofenac* help to ease pain by reducing inflammation, so an understanding of inflammation is required before we can be confident that we know precisely how these drugs work. Again, there are plenty of (often very heavy) pathology books in the library but by now we have accumulated quite a pile of textbooks from which to study the subject of pharmacology. We have our anatomy and physiology textbook, our pathology textbook and finally our pharmacology textbook.

Do I really need all these textbooks?

Fortunately – no! *Introducing Pharmacology* has been specially written for the reader without a background in physiology, pathology and pharmacology. In its 11 chapters, *Introducing Pharmacology* covers most of the commonly prescribed drugs and explains their action relative to the physiology and pathology of the system concerned. Naturally, as you progress in your studies, you will need to refer to more advanced textbooks and journals but you should be able to obtain a sound understanding of the basics of the subject here.

Introducing Pharmacology is divided into two parts:

In **Part 1** we look at the fundamentals of pharmacology, taking you down among the cells to the (mainly) protein structures targeted by drugs. We also look at how the body processes and eliminates the drugs that have been administered; this will help you to understand why some drugs can be given in tablet form while others need to be injected. You are no doubt aware that most drugs have the potential to cause side-effects or to interact with other drugs, and in Part 1 we explore how this happens.

In **Part 2**, when you have read Part 1 and have a good grasp of the fundamentals of pharmacology, we can then proceed to learn how individual drugs produce their therapeutic (and sometimes unwanted) effects on the body. We have divided Part 2 into chapters that are devoted to the major drug groups as used for specific organ systems – circulatory, respiratory, digestive system, etc. These chapters will follow a common format that will, firstly, examine the basic anatomy and physiology of the organ system. Secondly, the chapter will look at key pathologies that affect the system – for example, asthma in the respiratory system and high blood pressure in the circulatory system. Finally, when you are sure that you understand the physiology and pathology, we will examine the key drugs used to treat those pathologies.

As *Introducing Pharmacology* is an introductory textbook, it covers primarily those drugs that you will encounter regularly in general clinical practice. Some drugs are rarely found outside specialist areas such as operating theatres or cancer wards, and to keep the book to its remit of *introducing pharmacology*, these more specialist drugs have been omitted. However, all drugs have similarities in their modes of action, so by reading this book and understanding the basic principles of pharmacology, you should have the knowledge necessary to access more advanced publications dealing with these specialist drugs.

As you read each chapter, you will find a few special features that help to keep you involved in the learning process and also ensure that you have understood what you have just read.

WHERE ARE WE STARTING FROM?

This provides a few short questions to test your background knowledge before you start a chapter. Answers are provided at the end of the chapter.

ONE SMALL QUESTION

This character pops up frequently and asks those awkward questions that keep us on our toes.

DID YOU KNOW

These are interesting snippets of information relating to the text that may broaden your understanding of a particular topic.

IN PRACTICE

These are notes that help you to apply your understanding of pharmacology to clinical practice.

REALITY CHECK

It is easy to read something and think that it makes sense, but have you really understood it? This feature prompts you to stop for a second and consider.

KEY FACT

Highlights important concepts or ideas.

ANOTHER WAY TO PICTURE THIS

Sometimes pharmacological concepts can be quite difficult to grasp, but by using an analogy from everyday experience they can make more sense.

CASE STUDY

These mini case studies appear in Part 2 and relate to the drugs and diseases you are exploring in that chapter. You are encouraged to think about what you have learned and apply that knowledge to practice.

A QUICK RECAP

Highlights the key concepts and ideas that you have been reading about over the previous few pages.

RUNNING WORDS

At the end of each chapter there is a list of all of the technical terms that have appeared in that chapter. Check them one by one and tick them off when you are certain you understand them.

YOUR TURN TO TRY

Now you have finished the chapter, you can test yourself with these mini-quizzes to find out how much you have learned and remembered. Answers are provided at the end of the book.

This book has been written primarily for the reader with little or no previous knowledge of the subject of pharmacology and perhaps may not have studied anatomy and physiology in any great depth. Hopefully, you should find *Introducing Pharmacology* accessible and understandable. The book has been written in an informal manner but without sacrificing scientific accuracy. In a society where the text message and e-mail are the preferred methods of communication, many readers are put off by a formal, dry academic style of writing that is the norm in many textbooks, but there is no reason why science cannot be communicated effectively in a language that everyone understands. Of course there are long words and technical terms that have to be learned because those are the words and terms that are used and understood by fellow professionals. This does not mean that we cannot communicate in plain English without resorting to jargon or 'in-house' acronyms that are only understood by the initiated few. In *Introducing Pharmacology* you will find plenty of case studies, clinical notes and self-test questions that break up the narrative into manageable sections. When you have finished working through the book you should have a good grasp of the basics of the subject, the key specialist terms used in pharmacology and be ready to move onto the next stage of applying what you have learned to your clinical practice.

So, find a nice new pad of A4 paper, sharpen your pencil and get ready for some interesting (if occasionally challenging) pharmacology.

A brief note about the drug names used in this book

The drugs in *Introducing Pharmacology* use the Recommended International Non-proprietary Names (rINN) from the European Pharmacopoeia which are replacing the British Approved Names (BAN). Some of these might be slightly different from what you currently encounter in clinical practice so, for example, **phenobarbital** replaces **phenobarbitone**, **furosemide** replaces **frusemide** and **lidocaine** replaces **lignocaine**. The rINN names are the names that appear in the *British National Formulary* (BNF) and are becoming the accepted form in UK practice.

As is standard for most pharmacology books, *Introducing Pharmacology* uses the generic (rINN) names for drugs rather than the proprietary or trade names. The generic names refer to a standardised formula for that particular drug, whereas the manufacturer's proprietary or trade name describes the formulation of the drug supplied by that particular manufacturer. For example, *fluoxetine* is the generic name of Prozac® which is the name given to *fluoxetine* by its manufacturer – Eli Lilly & Co Ltd. *Salbutamol* is the generic name for Ventolin® produced by GlaxoSmithKline plc. Although some proprietary names may be better known than the generic names, *Introducing Pharmacology* generally uses the generic names because some drugs, especially those that are out of copyright, may have many proprietary versions produced by various manufacturers and it would be impossible to use them all or decide which among them was the best-known name. In *Introducing Pharmacology*, the generic name is indicated by the name being highlighted in *italicised bold* letters.

Introducing Pharmacology and clinical practice

While you will find the study of pharmacology very useful and relevant to your clinical practice, it is not strictly a clinical subject and *Introducing Pharmacology* will not be imparting clinical advice. Case studies are included in Part 2 of this book solely to demonstrate the relevance of pharmacology to practice. The decision about which drug to administer to which patient at which dose, at which time and by which route is a clinical decision that requires expertise acquired in clinical practice and clinical training.

Roger McFadden

Acknowledgements

Above all, the author would like to acknowledge the assistance, support and forbearance of Nicola Peterson (the Lady-wife) who has tirelessly and without complaint, proof-read and corrected innumerable drafts of this book. Her advice has been invaluable and her perceptive (and interesting) ideas on punctuation have added greatly to the enjoyment of the writing process!

Additionally, the author would like to thank colleagues from the Faculty of Health at Birmingham City University for their support and advice. These include; Lilieth Williams, Pat James, Simon Dobbs, Imran Khan, Bridget Malkin, Gary O'Grady and Jim Chapman.

Part 1

Principles of pharmacology

Chapter 1

Let's start at basics: Cells and how they work

AIMS

By the time you have finished the chapter you should be able to understand:

1 The structure and function of cells (cells are the prime target for most drugs)
2 Some basic biochemistry (drugs mostly target biochemical processes in cells).

CONTENTS

Introduction

Pharmacology can be quite daunting to the student approaching the subject for the first time. The reason for this is that most pharmacological activity takes place at a cellular or biochemical level and relatively few people are really comfortable down among the cells and molecules. However, this is the level where we need to be, not only to understand the subject of pharmacology but also to understand the literature relating to the subject. This literature is not just textbooks on pharmacology but the clinical reference books such as the **British National Formulary** (BNF) that you will find in daily use in every UK hospital ward and GP surgery. The BNF appears in an updated edition at six-monthly intervals and is published jointly by the British Medical Association and the Royal Pharmaceutical Society of Great Britain. Clinical practitioners use this standard reference book on licensed drugs to ensure that the drug they are prescribing is suitable for the patient, that the patient is being prescribed the correct dose and that the drug will not interact with other drugs. However, a look at the contents page of the BNF will quickly convince you that you need to have some understanding of pharmacology, just to access and use this book. Here is a short sample of the section headings relating to various classes of drugs contained in the BNF:

- Calcium channel blockers
- Selective beta-2 agonists
- Angiotensin-converting enzyme inhibitors
- Alpha-adrenoceptor blocking drugs
- Non-steroidal anti-inflammatory drugs
- H_2 receptor antagonists
- Selective serotonin re-uptake inhibitors
- Cyclo-oxygenase-2 inhibitors

If you already understand these terms then you can probably progress quickly to a more advanced pharmacology book. However, if you do not understand the terms then you will need to learn them – especially if you are going to be involved either in the prescribing or the administration of drugs to patients. You not only need to be familiar with the terms but you also need to know what the terms mean – which is a fundamental requirement to ensure patient safety. Nursing staff who administer drugs to patients are responsible for the safe administration of those drugs. This means that those staff must be familiar with those drugs, how they work in the body, how they may cause side-effects and possibly interact with other drugs. The classes of drugs mentioned above are in fact the clinical names of some of the most common drug groups that include **antihypertensives**, **analgesics**, **bronchodilators** and **antidepressants**.

One of the key aims of *Introducing Pharmacology* is to familiarise you with the language of pharmacology, the names of drugs and the terms that you will find on every packet of drugs and in every publication dealing with the clinical use of those drugs. You will need this language not only to study and understand pharmacology but also to discuss drugs and their effects with patients and fellow professionals.

WHERE ARE WE STARTING FROM?

Normally at this point – at the beginning of a chapter – we start with a short quiz to see how much you already know about a particular topic. However, as this is the first chapter of *Introducing Pharmacology*, we will assume that your knowledge of the subject is limited to what you read about drugs in the newspaper and hear about them on the radio and TV. For some future chapters you will need to do some background reading, but at this stage we are assuming that you are entirely new to the subject. We will therefore start at the best place – the beginning!

1.1   Levels of organisation: from cells to systems

Drugs are chemicals that are introduced into the human body to treat or prevent disease. Drugs can relieve symptoms such as pain and swelling, resolve problems such as indigestion and anxiety or manage problems such as heart disease. There are hundreds of different types of drugs designed to treat hundreds of disorders and each type of drug works by a unique action of its own. The way that some drugs work is relatively straightforward while others have quite complex actions. Ultimately, however, if we are going to understand how any of these drugs work, we need to transport ourselves to the level at which most drugs work – the cell.

What exactly is a cell?

Good question – we will examine cells in some detail later in this chapter. At the moment you just need to know that cells are very small structures that form the building blocks of tissues and organs.

Now, although the basic action of most drugs can be explained at a cellular level, they eventually have an effect on organs and systems that can be observed either by the clinical practitioner or by the patient. This means that to really understand the action of drugs you have to be able to connect their action at cellular level with their effect on organs and systems. Let us illustrate this by looking at some common drugs and drug groups with which you are probably familiar (or at least have heard of) – see Table 1.1. All of these drugs act on specific cells of the body but have an effect above cellular level.

The gap between target cell and the effect the drug has on the body is highlighted in the table by an arrow and this is largely what pharmacology is about – explaining how a drug that targets a particular cell produces its therapeutic effect on the body. To understand this, you need to appreciate that the body has various levels of organisation.

Table 1.1 Some common drugs, their cellular targets and their effects

Drug	Cell target	Mechanism	Therapeutic effects
Beta-blockers	Heart cells	→	Prevents an increase in heart rate
Local anaesthetics	Nerve cells	→	Prevents pain in minor surgery
Analgesics	Immune cells	→	Reduces inflammatory pain
Antidepressants	Nerve cells	→	Relieves depression
Statins	Liver cells	→	Reduces blood cholesterol levels

We divide the human body into levels of organisation for much the same reason as we divide a book into sections and chapters – it helps us to understand the structure better. Figure 1.1 shows a simplified hierarchy of structures, starting with cell chemistry and moving upwards to the whole body. As an example of this hierarchy we have used the circulatory system, but bear in mind that this simplified diagram does not imply that the heart is made up of only one type of tissue. There may be only one heart but it is made up of several different types of tissue and these tissues are made up of their own specialised types of cells.

Most drugs interact initially with the first two categories, cell **organelles** and their components, the chemicals of which they are made. However, the effects of drugs are generally observed on the body as a whole or the organ systems. For example, the anti-angina drug *glyceryl trinitrate* (GTN) targets the cells of

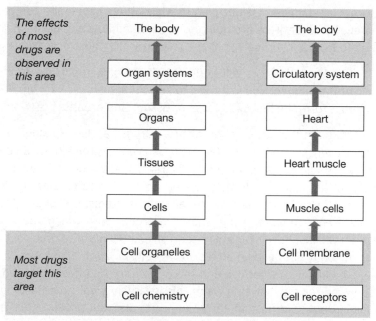

Figure 1.1 Levels of organisation within the human body. The hierarchy of organisation of the heart and circulatory system is given as an example.

various blood vessels, including those of the heart itself, but the effect observed by the patient is the lessening of his or her chest pain. Another example is the antihypertensive drug *verapamil*, which reduces blood pressure by targeting the cell membrane of heart muscle cells. Here the effect is on the circulatory system where you will observe a fall in blood pressure.

In Part 2 of *Introducing Pharmacology* we will be following the stories of most of our major drug groups from their interaction with cells right through to their therapeutic effect on organs systems. You will see that when we take each stage a step at a time, then pharmacology is actually quite a straightforward subject and is nowhere near as daunting as it may at first seem. But first things first – we need to familiarise ourselves with cells and some of the basic biochemistry that takes place in those cells.

1.2   A brief introduction to cells

Most drugs bind to proteins and most of these proteins are found in and on cells. Those proteins that form the targets for drugs are explored in more detail in Chapter 2, but in the meantime we need to find out a bit more about cells and the proteins they produce.

Cells and cell components

Cells are the building blocks that make up most tissues and our bodies contain trillions of cells. Most cells are specialised to a particular task. For example, muscle cells contract, nerve cells conduct nervous impulses and glandular cells secrete hormones. Drugs interact with these specialised cells and the effects of these interactions will be discussed in detail in the second part of *Introducing Pharmacology* when we look at the major drug groups. However, although these cells may look very different on the outside and each may have its own specialised function, inside they are fairly similar. A few cells such as muscle cells contain special proteins that enable them to contract, but otherwise cells have many internal features in common. To understand the principles of how drugs work on cells, it is necessary to have a basic understanding of cells, their structure and what goes on inside them. Figure 1.2 is a diagram of a typical cell.

The components of cells: organelles

It is important that we do not think of cells simply as the building blocks of tissues because in reality they are miniature wonderlands of biochemical activity. Every second in every cell there are thousands upon thousands of biochemical reactions taking place to maintain the cell and also to enable it to perform its task as part of a community of cells that makes up our tissues and organs. If you look at a cell through a good-quality, high-powered microscope, you can see that

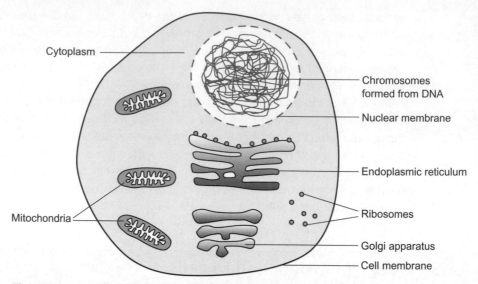

Figure 1.2 A typical human cell showing the principal organelles.

it contains many small structures. These are called the **organelles** (literally small organs) and are common to all cells. Each organelle has a specific function.

Several organelles are involved in the production of proteins. These are the **nucleus**, the **endoplasmic reticulum**, the **Golgi apparatus** and the **ribosomes**. Tens of thousands of different proteins are made by cells and, as mentioned previously, proteins are the main target for drugs. **Mitochondria** are small, bean-shaped organelles that produce most of the energy for the cell. They use the energy from fuel such as glucose and lipid to produce **adenosine triphosphate** (ATP), a small packet of energy that powers most of the cell's biochemical processes. You will need to understand more about ATP because some drugs target structures and mechanisms that use ATP. The process whereby our cells make ATP is quite complex, but we need to have a basic knowledge of the process because some diseases such as angina affect energy production and some drugs such as *glyceryl trinitrate* help to maintain the body's ability to make ATP. This process is called **cellular respiration** and we will examine it in more detail later in this chapter.

- **Cytoplasm.** This is basically the contents of the cell. It is composed of the organelles and the **cytosol**, a semitransparent solution of enzymes, nutrients and electrolytes, necessary for the myriad of processes that take place continuously in each cell.

- **Cell membrane.** This important structure is a thin membrane that encloses the contents of our cells and separates them from the **extracellular fluid** outside the cell. The cell membrane regulates what goes into and out of the cell. It is composed mainly of a **phospholipid bilayer** interspersed with **cholesterol** and it is incredibly thin, around 7 nanometres (1 nanometre is 1,000,000th of 1 millimetre). The components of the bilayer are arranged as shown in Figure 1.3.

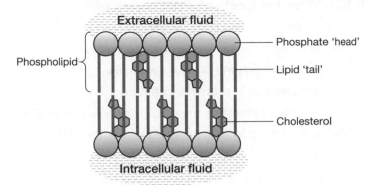

Figure 1.3 The phospholipid bilayer makes up the cell membrane. Cholesterol molecules within the bilayer help to stabilise it.

The phosphate heads are **hydrophilic** (attracted to water) so they happily sit in the watery environment of the extracellular fluid outside the cell and the **intracellular** fluid inside the cell. The lipid tails are **hydrophobic** (repelled by water) and form a stable layer in the water-free environment between the outer and inner layer of phosphate heads. Cholesterol molecules give the structure additional stability. There are proteins embedded in the cell membrane that have a variety of roles. These proteins include **receptors, ion channels, enzymes** and **carrier proteins**. As mentioned at the beginning of the chapter, proteins are the main targets for therapeutic drugs and these four proteins are our key targets.

Intracellular relates to that which is within the cell and **extracellular** is that which is outside the cell.

A section of cell membrane might look like that shown in Figure 1.4.

KEY FACT

Many drugs bind to the cell membrane, either to receptors, ion channels, enzymes or carrier proteins. Not all enzymes are attached to membranes, others may be found inside or outside cells and these also may be the target of drugs.

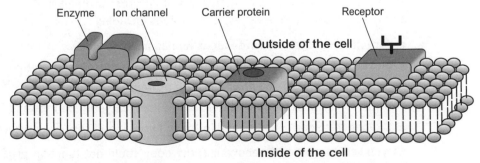

Figure 1.4 A section of a cell membrane showing various membrane proteins.

A QUICK RECAP on the function of cell organelles

- Nucleus – contains DNA that codes for our proteins.
- Endoplasmic reticulum – is involved in protein synthesis.
- Golgi apparatus – is involved in protein synthesis.
- Ribosomes – are involved in protein synthesis.
- Mitochondria – produces most of the cell's energy in the form of ATP.
- Cell membrane – controls what enters and leaves the cell.

1.3 A brief introduction to (basic) biochemistry

Biochemistry is where biology and chemistry meet; it is basically the chemistry of biological processes. Most people, when they think of chemistry, conjure up images of scientists in white coats doing experiments in laboratories full of strange smells and bubbling test-tubes. Biochemistry labs are very similar except the materials in the test-tubes are of biological origin such as enzymes and lipids. Biochemistry, as with all subjects, can be quite challenging if studied in depth. Fortunately, you can learn the essentials, certainly enough for basic clinical pharmacology, without too much chemistry – and not an equation in sight.

Do I really need to learn this biochemistry?

Yes, unfortunately you do. Drugs target many biochemical processes that take place in and around cells. For example, most drugs target proteins, so you need to know what proteins are. Some antibacterial drugs target protein synthesis, so you need to understand this process. Statins are a common group of drugs that lower cholesterol, so you need to understand lipids.

Protein and protein synthesis

Drugs target proteins, but before we look at how the cells make protein, it may be useful to ask ourselves: 'What is protein?'

Proteins are an important and probably the most variable class of biological molecules. There are tens of thousands of different proteins in the human body and they perform a wide variety of functions including . . .

- Structure – proteins form tendons and ligaments
- Movement – proteins found in muscles produce muscle contraction
- Communication – many hormones are proteins
- Defence – **antibodies** that attack and destroy bacteria are proteins
- **Oxygen** transport – **haemoglobin** found in red blood cells is a protein

As you can see from the above list, the body could not function properly without proteins. Not included in this list are the four protein targets for most of our

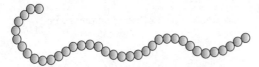

Figure 1.5 Chains of amino acids make up a protein. The sequence of the amino acids and the length of the chain largely determine the character of the protein.

drugs – ion channels, enzymes, receptors and carrier proteins. These are quite specialised types of protein and are found mainly in and on cells. In Chapter 2 we will explore each of them in some depth.

Proteins are made of chains of **amino acids** (small nitrogen-containing molecules) – Figure 1.5. There are 20 different types of amino acid in human protein and we obtain these amino acids from our food. Meat, fish, eggs, nuts and beans are foods that are rich in protein and consequently rich in amino acids. The digestive system breaks down the protein in these foods into its component amino acids, which we then absorb into the body for our cells to reassemble into human protein.

The nature of the protein is largely determined by the length of the chain and the order of the amino acids. Another factor characteristic of each individual protein is the way the chain of amino acids folds into its final three-dimensional shape. Some are long and thin such as the structural protein **collagen** found in tendons, and these are called **filamentous proteins**. Others form a more rounded, globular shape such as the oxygen-carrying protein **haemoglobin**, and these are naturally called **globular proteins**.

ANOTHER WAY TO PICTURE THIS

You can think of amino acids rather like letters in the alphabet. There are an infinite number of words that can be formed, each word's individual character being determined by its length and the order of its letters. Similarly, there are an infinite number of proteins that could be made, determined by the length and sequence of the chain of amino acids.

The body's cells all have the ability to make over 20,000 different proteins, the difference determined by the length and sequence of the amino acids in the chain. This means that inside each cell there needs to be a code or instruction to ensure that when the cell makes a particular protein, the amino acids are in the correct sequence and the chain is of the correct length. This code for our proteins is contained within **DNA** (**deoxyribose nucleic acid**), an incredibly thin ribbon-like molecule that is found in the nucleus of each cell. There are 46 lengths of DNA in all human cells (except the sperm and egg which each have 23) and each length of DNA is called a **chromosome**. Although individual cells do not need to make every kind of protein, each cell contains the codes for every one of our 20,000 or so proteins. How the cell knows which proteins to make and when to make them is not fully understood.

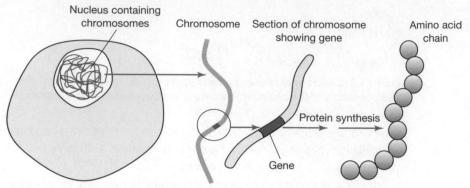

Figure 1.6 Proteins are produced from information contained in chromosomes. The information coded in each gene is translated into the correct sequence of amino acids by a process called protein synthesis.

The piece of DNA that codes for a single chain of amino acids or protein is called a **gene** (Figure 1.6). There are over 30,000 genes that code for the 20,000+ proteins that cells make. There are more genes than proteins because some proteins such as haemoglobin are made up of more than one amino acid chain and so need more than one gene to code for each chain.

Some proteins are used within the cell and others are exported from the cell for use in other parts of the body. Many proteins are lodged in the cell membrane such as receptors, ion channels, enzymes or carrier proteins. These are the key drug targets that are examined in Chapter 2. Proteins come in many shapes and sizes and perform many functions. Enzymes are among the most numerous types of protein; they are complex structures that take part in most of the body's biochemical reactions and are also a major target for drugs.

DID YOU KNOW . . . that every cell contains around 2 metres of DNA? There are well over a trillion cells in the human body, so the total length of DNA must be at least 2 billion kilometres, which is more than enough to stretch from the Earth to the Sun over 10 times!!!

How cells make proteins

When a cell needs to make a protein there follows a complex process that involves finding the correct gene and translating the instructions contained in that gene into a protein with the correct sequence of amino acids, a chain of the appropriate length and folded into the correct shape. The process involves cooperation between several organelles in the cell: the nucleus obviously, as it contains the chromosomes that carry the code in their genes; the ribosomes that are responsible for the assembly of the amino acids into a chain that will make up the protein; and finally the endoplasmic reticulum and Golgi apparatus that fold the protein into its final shape.

Lipids

Lipids are an important group of molecules. As well as being a good source of energy and providing insulation from the cold, they are the building blocks of some hormones and also form a significant part of cell membranes. As most drugs target proteins in the cell membranes, you will need a basic understanding of lipids in order to understand the nature of the cell membrane and ultimately the action of drugs.

There are many different types of lipid but they can initially be divided into two groups . . .

- oils – these are liquid at room temperature

- fats – these are solid at room temperature.

Oils are generally obtained from plants and fish whereas fats are generally obtained from meat such as beef and pork. We can obtain these fats from the natural foods we eat but a good proportion of our lipid intake is from processed products such as cooking oils, margarine, butter and cheese.

Triglycerides, also known as **triacylglycerols**, are an important group of lipids and most of the lipids that we eat and store in the body are triglycerides. Their structure is relatively simple, just three long **fatty acid** chains joined to a glycerol molecule (Figure 1.7).

Fatty acids come in various forms and you may have seen their names on the labels of some processed foods. Most of these names refer to the ratio and arrangement of carbon and hydrogen atoms in the fatty acid chains. We will just mention them here so you will understand what they do, but we will not go any deeper into their biochemistry.

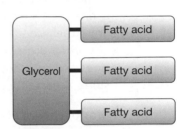

Figure 1.7 Triglycerides are composed of three fatty acid chains attached to a glycerol molecule.

- **Saturated fatty acids** – mainly found in animal fats and processed foods.

- **Mono-unsaturated fatty acids** – only vegetable in origin, for example olive oil.

- **Polyunsaturated fatty acids** – only vegetable in origin, for example sunflower oil.

The type and balance of the lipids we consume in our diet has important implications for our health, especially the health of our heart. We are currently recommended to consume less saturated fat and use more mono-unsaturated oils, such as olive oil, in preference.

Cholesterol is a sterol lipid that is predominantly made in the liver, but it is also obtained from animal products such as eggs. It is an important substance because it stabilises our cell membranes and is also a component of **bile**, a digestive product made in the liver and secreted into the **duodenum** via the **bile duct**. Cholesterol is also the raw material for steroid hormones such as **oestrogen**, **testosterone** and **vitamin D**. Cholesterol regulation is important because, if it gets out of balance, it can encourage cardiovascular disease. Various drugs such as statins are widely prescribed to reduce cholesterol levels.

> **DID YOU KNOW . . .** that vitamin D is actually a steroid hormone rather than a vitamin? It is made in the skin when exposed to sunlight but is also obtained in the diet from fatty fish such as sardines and herring. Many foods such as breakfast cereals are fortified with vitamin D. A shortage of vitamin D can cause rickets in children.

Carbohydrates and sugars

Just as a car needs fuel to keep it going, the body also needs fuel to provide the energy for the thousands of biochemical reactions that take place every second. We get the energy primarily from **carbohydrates** in the form of **starches** and **sugars** but lipids also make an important contribution to our energy needs. There are no drugs that have sugars and starches as their prime targets, but these substances play an important role in the body. As some drugs such as *insulin* have a direct effect on glucose metabolism, you need a basic familiarity with this important group of molecules.

Carbohydrates can be divided into three groups: **monosaccharides**, **disaccharides** and **polysaccharides**. As 'saccharide' means sugar, these three groups are single sugars, double sugars and multiple sugars respectively.

Monosaccharides

These are single sugars that include **glucose, fructose** and **galactose**. Glucose is one of the most common monosaccharides as it forms the building blocks of polysaccharides such as **starch, glycogen** and **cellulose**. Glucose is a key fuel for human metabolism which is why we need a good supply of carbohydrates for our daily energy requirement. There is very little free glucose in nature and it is generally found as disaccharides or, more commonly, polysaccharides such as starch. Our digestive systems contain enzymes that break down the disaccharides and polysaccharides into energy-rich monosaccharide glucose molecules. These are transported in the blood to the cells of the body where the glucose is broken down to release its energy to power biochemical processes.

Disaccharides

These are two monosaccharides joined together. Common disaccharides include maltose, sucrose and lactose. The sugar that we put in our tea and coffee is sucrose, a disaccharide composed of glucose and fructose.

Polysaccharides

These are long chains of monosaccharides joined together. Common glucose-based polysaccharides include **starch, glycogen** and **cellulose**.

Starch is a **polymer** (chain) of glucose molecules that is produced in plants. It is a major source of fuel for humans. Potatoes, wheat and rice contain large amounts of starch and so are important energy-rich foods for us. Starch is broken down into disaccharides and finally into individual glucose molecules by enzymes in the digestive system.

Glycogen is a polymer of glucose found in animal cells, stored especially in the liver and skeletal muscle. When the cells require energy, enzymes break down glycogen into glucose molecules. Glucose released by the liver cells can be used to top-up the glucose in the blood when circulating levels are low.

Cellulose is similar in structure to starch, except for a small biochemical difference that makes it impossible for humans to digest. This is unfortunate because it is a major structural component of plants and the most abundant form of glucose on the planet. Its indigestible nature does confer some benefits because it increases the bulk of our food and provides the fibre necessary for a healthy digestion. Animals such as cows, that get their energy from grass, rely on bacteria in their digestive systems to break down the cellulose into glucose.

A QUICK RECAP on proteins, lipids and sugars

- There are many thousands of different proteins in the body.
- Proteins are key targets for drugs.
- DNA in the nucleus of cells codes for our proteins.
- The section of DNA that codes for one protein is called a gene.
- Lipids are an important source of energy and are also components of cell membranes.
- Carbohydrates are an important source of energy, especially in the form of glucose.

Cellular respiration and the production of ATP

Cells need energy to perform many of their functions and an example of cells that need plenty of energy is the muscle cells. These cells contract and, in the case of skeletal muscle cells, work in groups to contract whole muscles that allow us to engage in sporting activities such as running, tennis and cycling. We can expend a lot of energy when engaged in these sports and this energy comes from the adenosine triphosphate (ATP) produced in every cell of the body. There is a fundamental law of physics that (put simply) says that energy can be transferred but not created; therefore, in the case of cells, there needs to be a source of energy that enables them to produce ATP. This energy is obtained primarily from glucose in energy-rich foods we eat, especially the starchy foods such as rice, potatoes and wheat. Triglycerides from the lipids found in animal and plant products also make a significant contribution to our energy requirements.

> **DID YOU KNOW**...that in some extreme sports, athletes can burn over 30,000 kJ of energy in one day – that is four times as much as the average person? In the *Tour de France*™ cycle race, some stages are over 200 km and it has been calculated that riders would need to eat over 25 cheeseburgers each day to top-up their energy!

ATP is produced in every cell of the body because every cell needs energy to perform its numerous biochemical reactions, and the original source of this energy is either glucose or lipids. However, these are large molecules and while they contain plenty of energy, that energy is not in a usable form for most biochemical reactions. As cells need small packets of energy, they break down glucose and lipids by a gradual process into their component parts and during this process energy is released and transferred to ATP.

> **KEY FACT**
>
> All cells need energy in the form of ATP. They use the energy from glucose and lipids to make their ATP.

Adenosine triphosphate (ATP) is part of a family of molecules that also includes **adenosine diphosphate** (ADP). If you think of ATP as a small rechargeable battery, it is uncharged in the ADP form and fully charged in the ATP form (Figure 1.8). The biochemical process in the cell that charges ADP into ATP is called **cellular respiration**.

When ATP has performed its task, perhaps activating an enzyme or moving ions across a membrane, it loses much of its energy and becomes low-energy ADP which must then return to the mitochondria to be recharged into ATP (Figure 1.9).

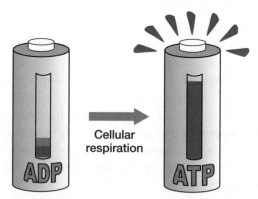

Figure 1.8 Comparing the cell's energy molecule to a rechargeable battery. Cellular respiration charges ADP to its energy-packed form of ATP.

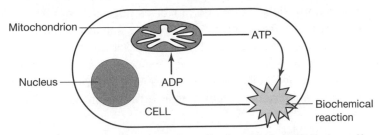

Figure 1.9 ADP is recharged in the mitochondria to ATP that can then power biochemical reactions in the cell. When it gives up its energy, ATP becomes ADP that returns to the mitochondria to be recharged again into ATP.

The process that recharges ADP to ATP is called cellular respiration, which is a fundamental process common to all animals and plants. Cellular respiration is at the heart of our metabolism; it explains why we breathe, why we are warm-blooded animals and why we eat the energy-rich foods we all enjoy. This process takes place in every cell of our body and can be described by a simple word formula:

Carbohydrate / Lipids + Oxygen ⟶ ATP + Carbon dioxide + Water + Heat

Energy production is all about the ATP that maintains our body's metabolism and therefore life itself. Basically the formula says that in the presence of **oxygen** the body can use energy-rich foods such as carbohydrate and lipids to energise ADP into ATP. In the process, waste products such as **carbon dioxide**, water and heat are produced.

The oxygen that is essential for this process is obtained from the air that we breathe and transported in the blood from the lungs to the cells of the body (Figure 1.10). Carbon dioxide, the waste gas produced in cellular respiration, is transported in the opposite direction, from the cells to the lungs where it is exhaled into the atmosphere.

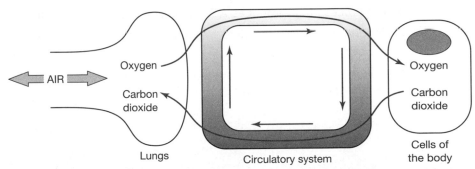

Figure 1.10 Simplified diagram showing the transport of respiratory gasses between the lungs and the body's cells. Oxygen carried into the lungs from the air we breathe is transported to the cells via the blood. The waste gas, carbon dioxide, is transported in the opposite direction, from the cells to the lungs where it is breathed out into the atmosphere.

The process of cellular respiration involves dozens of enzymes that work in complex pathways to break down carbohydrates and lipids to form ATP. Oxygen is essential for the efficiency of this process and if any disease reduces the supply of oxygen to cells and tissues then the consequences can be very serious indeed: without oxygen, cells cannot produce ATP, and without ATP cells die. This is what happens when someone has a heart attack or stroke – as we will see later in Chapter 4.

IN PRACTICE

Any disease that affects the lungs can cause problems with gas exchange. Bronchitis and emphysema are very common chronic diseases of the lungs. Shortness of breath, wheezing and cough are common symptoms and lack of oxygen may cause cyanosis (a blue tinge to the lips and fingers).

As for the other waste products in this process, water simply diffuses into the tissues and mingles with the rest of the water in the body (don't forget we are composed of almost 65 per cent water). The heat produced in cellular respiration helps to keep our body warm with a core temperature steady, around 37°C.

REALITY CHECK

Can you now list the components of the word formula and explain where the oxygen and glucose/lipids come from. What happens to the carbon dioxide, water and heat?

A QUICK RECAP on cellular respiration

- Cells need energy for biochemical reactions.
- ATP is the source of energy for these biochemical reactions.
- The energy to produce ATP comes from energy-rich foods.
- The process that produces ATP is called cellular respiration.
- Cellular respiration requires oxygen that is transported from the lungs to the cells of the body.
- Cellular respiration produces carbon dioxide that is transported from the cells of the body to the lungs.

RUNNING WORDS

Here are some of the technical terms that were included in this chapter.
Read them one by one and tick them off when you are sure that you understand them.

ADP (adenosine diphosphate) p. 16
Amino acids p. 11
Analgesics p. 4
Antibodies p. 10
Antidepressants p. 4
Antihypertensives p. 4
ATP (adenosine triphosphate) p. 8
Bile p. 13
Bile duct p. 13
British National Formulary p. 4
Bronchodilators p. 4
Carbohydrates p. 14
Carbon dioxide p. 17
Carrier proteins p. 8
Cell membrane p. 8
Cellular respiration p. 8
Cellulose p. 14
Cholesterol p. 8
Chromosome p. 11
Collagen fibres p. 11

Cytoplasm p. 8
Cytosol p. 8
Deoxyribose nucleic acid (DNA) p. 11
Disaccharides p. 14
Duodenum p. 13
Endoplasmic reticulum p. 8
Enzymes p. 8
Extracellular fluid p. 8
Fatty acid p. 13
Filamentous proteins p. 11
Fructose p. 14
Galactose p. 14
Gene p. 12
Globular proteins p. 11
Glucose p. 14
Glycogen p. 14
Golgi apparatus p. 8
Haemoglobin p. 10
Hydrophilic p. 9
Hydrophobic p. 9
Intracellular fluid p. 8
Ion channels p. 8

Mitochondria p. 8
Mono-unsaturated (fat) p. 13
Monosaccharides p. 14
Nucleus p. 8
Oestrogen p. 13
Organelles p. 6
Oxygen p. 10
Phospholipid bilayer p. 8
Polymer p. 15
Polysaccharides p. 14
Polyunsaturated (fat) p. 13
Proteins p. 10
Receptors p. 8
Ribosomes p. 8
Saturated (fat) p. 13
Starches p. 14
Sugars p. 14
Testosterone p. 13
Triacylglycerols p. 13
Triglycerides p. 13
Vitamin D p. 13

REFERENCES AND FURTHER RECOMMENDED READING

All recommended websites are open access (but free registration is sometimes required).

British National Formulary (2008) BMJ Group and RPS Publishing.

British National Formulary Website – http://www.bnf.org/bnf/

Your turn to try

Now you have finished reading the first chapter it's time to find out how much you have learned and remembered. If you have not studied this area before, don't worry if you can't answer all of the questions. Reread the chapter and make sure that it all makes sense.

The answers to these questions are at the end of the book on page 283.

1 What is the (outline) function of the following cell organelles?
   (a) Nucleus
   (b) Ribosomes
   (c) Mitochondria
   (d) Cell membrane.

2 Is the cell membrane predominantly made of protein, lipid or carbohydrate?

3 Name the four principal protein targets for drugs.

4 What is the name for the section of DNA that codes for one protein?

5 What are the basic components of proteins?

6 What is the chemical difference between an oil and a fat?

7 What lipid is the raw material for steroid hormones?

8 What kind of polysaccharide is the main food source of energy for humans?

9 What two substances are required for efficient ATP production in humans?

10 What happens to the carbon dioxide produced in the process of cellular respiration?

Chapter 2

Protein targets for drugs

AIMS

By the time you have finished the chapter you will understand:

1 Why proteins make good targets for drugs
2 The structure of key protein targets for drugs
3 What happens when drugs bind to key protein targets.

CONTENTS

Introduction

In Chapter 1 we started our journey into the interesting if occasionally challenging world of pharmacology. We learned that cells are the prime target for most drugs and that those drugs mostly target biochemical processes in cells. This means that some knowledge of basic cell biology and biochemistry is absolutely essential to an understanding of pharmacology, and in this chapter we will start to apply that knowledge. Chapter 2 is where we start to examine the fundamental principles of pharmacology, where we will focus on the four key protein targets for drugs, namely receptors, ion channels, enzymes and carrier proteins. We will also encounter examples of specific drugs that interact with these protein targets and you should start to gain an insight into the basics of the subject and begin to feel more comfortable with the terminology relating to the cellular and biochemical world where most of our drugs exert their action. In the meantime, make sure that you work through this chapter carefully because the concept of protein targets underpins pharmacology and the terms we use here will appear throughout this book and in clinical manuals such as the *British National Formulary* (BNF), which you will encounter in almost every area of clinical practice.

WHERE ARE WE STARTING FROM?

This is the second chapter *of Introducing Pharmacology*, so we will assume that you have read the first chapter and now have an understanding of basic cell biology and biochemistry. You should know something about proteins, their basic structure and how they are made in cells. You should also understand how cells make their ATP in the process of cellular respiration.

Let's start off with a short quiz to enable you to check how much you remembered from Chapter 1.

1 Name the two principal components of the cell membrane.

_____

2 What process involves the nucleus, endoplasmic reticulum, Golgi apparatus and ribosomes?

_____

3 What are the basic components of protein?

_____

4 What do we call the length of DNA that codes for a protein?

_____

5 Mitochondria produce ATP. Fuel in the form of glucose or lipid is needed for this process, but what is the other essential component?

_____

6 Name the polymer of glucose that animal cells use to store their energy.

_____

Answers are at the end of the chapter on page 42.

How did you do? If you got most of the answers correct then you remembered most of the material you read in Chapter 1. Well done. If you only managed to answer one or two of the questions then it might be useful to read the first chapter again as these basic concepts will reappear regularly in the following chapters. Don't worry, however, because very few people can remember new material at the first reading. Persevere and it will become easier to assimilate as you get used to pharmacological concepts and scientific language.

2.1 Why do proteins make good targets for drugs?

As we saw in Chapter 1, most drugs target and bind to proteins, mostly on and in the cell membrane. These protein targets can be divided into four categories . . .

- Receptors
- Enzymes
- Ion channels
- Carrier proteins.

> **KEY FACT**
>
> Most drugs bind to proteins, specifically – ion channels, enzymes, receptors and carrier proteins.

Chapter 1 introduced us to proteins: what they are, what they do and how they are made. In this chapter we are going to examine the four categories of protein drug targets in some detail and will also meet examples of the drugs that target those proteins.

Drugs target and bind to proteins and, via a complex series of consequential events, this produces a therapeutic effect, perhaps reducing inflammation, relieving pain or lowering cholesterol levels etc. How the drugs produce these therapeutic effects will be explained in the second part of this book where we look at drug groups in more detail. First, however, we must ask ourselves why it is that proteins make such good targets for drugs.

Proteins make good targets for drugs for the three reasons detailed below.

1 There are many different types of protein

Proteins are incredibly varied in their structure. There are around 20,000 different proteins in the human body and each has its own particular task. This means that there are potentially around 20,000 different targets for drugs - although, in reality, only a small percentage of proteins are suitable targets. As most proteins are involved in tasks that are not linked to any particular disease, there is no point target-ing those proteins. Others are so crucial to normal cell function that it would be dangerous to target them with drugs. However, if only 1 per cent of those 20,000 plus proteins make a suitable target, then that gives us the 200 or so different types of drugs that appear in the BNF. Naturally there are many more drugs than this on the pharmacy shelves because different drug manufacturers often make their own version of a drug - especially if that particular drug is selling successfully.

2 Proteins have important roles in physiological processes

Proteins are also good targets because they are key players in every single physio-logical process. For example, circulation, respiration, nervous activity, renal function and immunity all depend on proteins. Interfere with a protein by targeting it with a drug and you will interfere with a physiological process. It is important to note, however, that targeting a protein could potentially have adverse effects on these physiological processes, so drug manufacturers need to ensure that the drugs they are developing will produce only the desired therapeutic effects. Very occasionally, manufacturers fail to realise that the drug they are developing has an unforeseen side-effect and in a few cases this has resulted in a drug being withdrawn.

3 Each organ and tissue has some protein distinctive to that organ and tissue

This means that if a drug targets that particular type of protein, it will exert an effect specifically on that particular organ or tissue. This is very important because we want our drugs to produce predictable results in tissues and organs where there are problems that need to be remedied. If an individual patient has a heart problem, we need a drug that targets the heart and only the heart. Because heart tissue has proteins found only in the heart, we can target those proteins and that specific organ. Similarly, if a patient has a bacterial infection, then we want a drug that kills bacterial cells but does not interfere with human body cells. Because some bacterial protein is substantially different from human protein, we can target the bacterial protein and not interfere with other proteins in the body.

Unfortunately, some proteins that make desirable targets for drugs are found on other organs and tissues, including some that have no involvement in the disease we are attempting to prevent or cure. This can cause problems because drugs can also bind to the proteins in those tissues and produce unwanted side-effects. We will explore this problem in more detail in Chapter 3.

A QUICK RECAP on why proteins make good targets for drugs

● There are many different proteins in many different tissues which gives us plenty of targets for our drugs.

● As proteins play key roles in physiological processes, they are worth targeting with drugs because, by doing so, we can influence those physiological processes.

● Different tissues express their own unique proteins, and drugs can therefore target those proteins and exert their effect specifically on those tissues.

● Some tissues express similar proteins to those being targeted and can become the targets themselves – resulting in side-effects.

2.2 Protein targets 1: receptors

Communication within the body is very important to ensure that it functions properly. Physiological processes with their myriad of tiny biochemical reactions must be coordinated to occur in the right place at the right time. One part of the brain needs to communicate with other parts of the brain and also with the organs and tissues under its control. Glands such as the pituitary and pancreas need to communicate with cells and tissues to ensure that the body's internal environment is kept stable – a process called **homeostasis**. Even adjacent cells need to communicate with each other so that they can work in cooperation to ensure that tissues function properly. All of this essential communication is effected by chemical messengers that are released from nerves, glands and a host of other cell types. These chemical messengers bind to receptors in and on other cells in the body to produce an effect in those target cells (Figure 2.1).

> **Homeostasis** is the name given to internal regulatory mechanisms that maintain steady-state physiological functions such as blood pressure, temperature and blood gas levels.

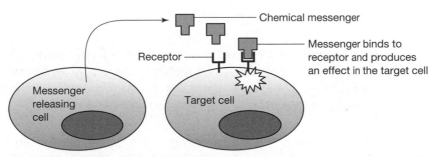

Figure 2.1 Chemical messengers released by a cell bind to receptors on an adjacent cell and produce an effect in that cell.

You may recall from Chapter 1 that the cell membrane is essentially lipid in structure and this prevents most chemicals (apart from lipids) from passing through it. This explains why many chemical messengers bind to the extracellular region of receptors embedded in the cell membrane. Some intracellular receptors are found within the cell and these are generally only targeted by steroid hormones and other lipid-based mediators that can pass through the cell membrane. Receptors are also very popular targets for drugs and we will devote the first part of this chapter to exploring how drugs interact with receptors.

Examples of some common drugs that interact with receptors include:

- *Salbutamol* – dilates the airways and relieves the symptoms of asthma
- *Atenolol* – slows the heart and relieves angina pain
- *Morphine* – inhibits pain pathways in the spinal cord to relieve severe pain
- *Doxazosin* – dilates peripheral blood vessels and reduces blood pressure.

Before we look in more detail at receptors, let us quickly examine some important chemical messengers that can broadly be divided into three groups – **hormones**, **neurotransmitters** and **mediators**. Many drugs mimic these chemical messengers so it is important to understand their function in order to understand how those drugs work.

Hormones are chemicals released by glandular tissue into the bloodstream. These chemicals circulate in the bloodstream and from there pass into tissues where they bind to cell receptors and produce an effect in those cells. The effect depends on the type of receptor and the type of cell. For example, when the hormone **insulin**, which is released by the pancreas, binds to an insulin receptor on a cell, it causes that cell to increase its uptake of glucose from the blood. The stress hormone **adrenaline** binds to adrenaline receptors on many different tissues and produces various effects, such as widening the bronchioles and increasing the heart rate.

Neurotransmitters are chemicals released from the terminals of neurons (nerve cells). These chemicals bind to receptors on other cells or neurons and produce various effects. For example, **acetylcholine** released from a motor neuron and binding to an acetylcholine receptor on a muscle cell would cause that cell to contract. **Noradrenaline** released by a **sympathetic** neuron and binding to a noradrenaline receptor on an **arteriole** (small artery) would cause the arterial muscle cells, and thus the arteriole itself, to contract.

> **Sympathetic neurons** are nerve cells that form a division of the autonomic nervous system that controls homeostasis. It is counterbalanced by the **parasympathetic** division. Generally the sympathetic system is dominant during activity and stress while the parasympathetic system takes over when we are at rest.

Mediators are mostly locally acting chemicals that bind to receptors on adjacent or nearby cells and produce an effect. **Histamine** is an example of a mediator that binds to histamine receptors on the cells that line the stomach, stimulating those cells to release the hydrochloric acid that breaks down food particles in the process of digestion.

You may also find these natural chemical messengers being referred to as **endogenous ligands**. 'Endogenous' just means that they are produced within the body and a ligand (from the Latin *ligare*, to bind) is effectively a chemical messenger that binds to a receptor.

> **KEY FACT**
>
> Cells of the body have receptors for chemical messengers (also called **endogenous ligands**) such as hormones, neurotransmitters and mediators.

Why do chemical messengers bind to receptors?

Chemical messengers bind to receptors because the receptor is the appropriate shape for the chemical messenger to bind to it, just as the lock on your front door is the appropriate shape for your front door key. The chemical messengers produced by the body are exactly the right shape for their receptor target (Figure 2.2). This correctness of shape is called **specificity** and we will encounter this term later in the chapter when we discuss the interactions between drugs and receptors. The specificity of a chemical messenger for its receptor is predominantly due to shape – like the correct fit of a key to a lock – but this is enhanced by tiny electrical forces of attraction in the region of the receptor where the chemical messenger docks. However, as we are only 'introducing pharmacology', we will keep things simple and discuss the fit of the chemical messenger for its receptor only in terms of shape.

Here is your turn to see whether you can match a chemical messenger to its receptor. The real-life molecular structures of chemical messengers and receptors are rather complex, so we will continue with the analogy of keys and locks. Figure 2.3 shows three keys that may represent three different hormones. The three locks represent three different types of receptor, possibly found on different tissues or organs. Which key best fits into which receptor?

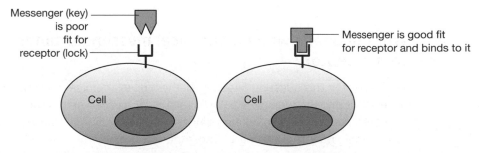

Figure 2.2 Only chemical messengers with a complementary shape to receptors will bind effectively to those receptors.

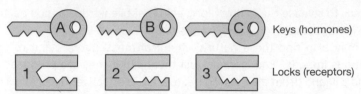

Figure 2.3 Match the key to its lock. (*Answers on page 42.*)

Why do drugs bind to receptors?

Drugs bind to receptors because the drug's molecular structure gives it a similar shape to that of the natural chemical messenger the body produces to target that receptor.

Here is an example: adrenaline binds to adrenaline receptors in the bronchioles of the lungs and causes bronchodilation (widening of the airways). As the drug *salbutamol* is similar in shape to adrenaline, it also binds to adrenaline receptors and produces the same effect as adrenaline, i.e. bronchodilation. Figure 2.4 shows the molecular structure of the hormone adrenaline and the drug *salbutamol*. You do not need a deep understanding of chemistry to observe the similarities in structure between the two molecules.

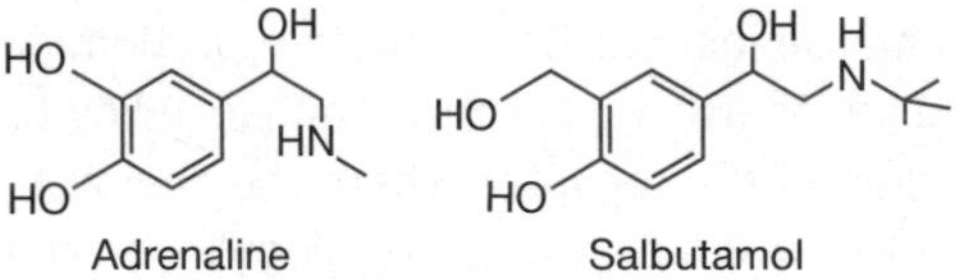

Adrenaline   Salbutamol

Figure 2.4 Adrenaline and *salbutamol* have similarities in molecular structure, so bind to the same receptors.

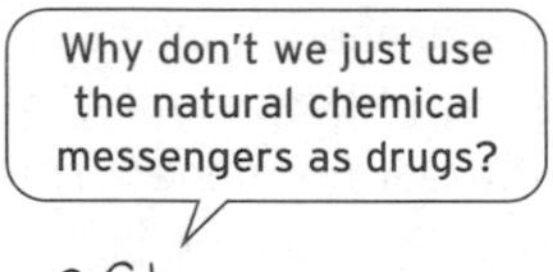

> Why don't we just use the natural chemical messengers as drugs?

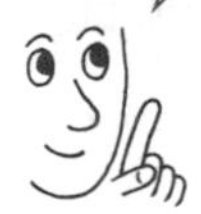

Good question. Sometimes we do. For example, adrenaline can be used as a drug when someone's blood pressure falls rapidly and the person goes into shock. However, relatively few natural chemical messengers make good drugs. We want drugs that are stable in storage, easy to administer and exert their therapeutic action over several hours or days. Few natural chemical messengers meet these criteria.

What happens when a chemical messenger binds to a receptor?

The answer to this question depends on the type of chemical messenger, the type of receptor and the type of cell. We have already touched on a few examples, such as insulin causing cells to take up glucose and acetylcholine causing muscle cells to contract. How the binding of these messengers to their receptors produces these effects is complex, involving intracellular biochemistry and is therefore beyond the scope of this introductory book. From the pharmacological viewpoint, however, the main imperative is to understand the overall effect on the cell or tissue – for example, when the messenger binds to its receptor, does it cause the cell or tissue to contract or relax, increase or decrease its activity, and so on?

What happens when a drug binds to a receptor?

A drug similar in shape to a natural chemical messenger will bind to the same receptor as that messenger – in fact, competing against the chemical messenger for the receptor site. How successfully it competes depends on the closeness of fit of the drug for the receptor – in other words, its specificity. Once a drug binds to a receptor it can do one of two things: it can either mimic the natural chemical messenger and produce the same effect as that chemical messenger, or bind to and block that receptor and produce no effect.

Drugs that are close enough in shape to the natural chemical messenger to bind to a receptor and produce the same effect as the original chemical messenger are termed **agonists**.

Drugs that are similar in shape to the original natural chemical messenger but bind to and block the receptor without producing a response are called **antagonists**, or sometimes just **blockers** – as in beta-blockers.

> **KEY FACT**
>
> **Agonist drugs** bind to receptors and mimic the effect of natural chemical messengers. **Antagonist drugs** bind to and block receptors from the effects of their natural chemical messengers.

Figure 2.5 shows a section of membrane with identical receptors for a natural chemical messenger which binds and produces an effect in the cell. Adjacent to it is an agonist drug that is quite similar in shape to the natural chemical messenger, binds to the receptor and produces the same effect. The antagonist drug has enough similarities in shape to the natural chemical messenger to bind to the receptor and block it but not enough to produce a response in the cell.

What's the point of a drug that blocks a receptor but produces no effect?

Good question. It may seem pointless to target a receptor without producing an effect but sometimes we want to prevent the effect that the natural chemical messenger produces. For example, adrenaline increases heart rate so by blocking adrenaline receptors with a beta-blocker we can keep heart rate down – very useful for angina sufferers.

Most drugs that bind to receptors have either an agonist or an antagonist action. We will come across many of these drugs in Part 2 of *Introducing Pharmacology*. As we have only just started to explore the subject, you may not be familiar with the names of agonist and antagonist drugs, so we will not provide a long list of examples. However, two drugs in common use that you may have encountered already are the bronchodilator *salbutamol* and the anti-angina beta-blocker *atenolol*.

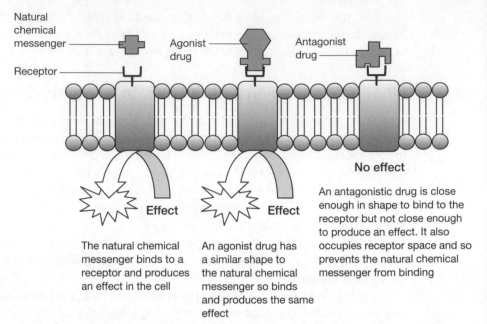

The natural chemical messenger binds to a receptor and produces an effect in the cell

An agonist drug has a similar shape to the natural chemical messenger so binds and produces the same effect

An antagonistic drug is close enough in shape to bind to the receptor but not close enough to produce an effect. It also occupies receptor space and so prevents the natural chemical messenger from binding

Figure 2.5 Agonist drugs mimic natural chemical messengers. They bind to their receptors and produce the same effect. Antagonist drugs bind to and block receptors, preventing the natural chemical messengers from binding.

- *Salbutamol* – an agonist for adrenaline receptors in the lungs. It stimulates the receptors and produces bronchodilation (opening of the airways) which helps to relieve asthma attacks.

- *Atenolol* – an antagonist for adrenaline receptors on the heart, blocks the receptors from the stimulating activity of adrenaline. This reduces the workload of the heart which is useful for those suffering from angina.

Both *salbutamol* and *atenolol* have similarities in structure to adrenaline, but whereas *salbutamol* binds to adrenaline receptors and mimics the effect of adrenaline, *atenolol* binds and blocks the receptors without producing any effect in its own right.

REALITY CHECK

Can you now explain the difference between the agonist and antagonist action of drugs and give one example of each?

Sub-classes of receptor available as drug targets

The observant reader may have noticed from the above account of the action of *salbutamol* and *atenolol* that these two drugs appear to interact with different tissues despite the fact that they both target adrenaline receptors. The reason for this is that there are different types of adrenaline receptor in the bronchioles of the lungs and on the heart. In the lungs we find **beta-1 adrenaline receptors** and on the heart we find **beta-2 adrenaline receptors**. These different types of receptor are frequently identified by Greek letters, such as α (alpha) and β (beta). Note also that the adrenaline receptor has a scientific name. The general term for a receptor that responds to adrenaline (a hormone) or its close relative, noradrenaline (a neurotransmitter), is **adrenergic** but you may also find the term **adrenoceptor** used quite frequently.

Different tissues may have different sub-classes of adrenergic receptor; for example, β_1 receptors on the heart and β_2 receptors in the lungs. There are other types of adrenergic receptor but currently the only other one of pharmacological importance is the α_1 receptor found on the arterioles. The fact that there are several types or sub-classes of adrenergic receptor is very important in pharmacology because drugs can be designed to target specific sub-classes of receptor and therefore target specific tissues.

KEY FACT

Drugs can be targeted at specific sub-classes of **receptors** that are found on specific tissues.

Other natural chemical messengers have receptor groups subdivided into various sub-classes of receptors, and these are shown in Table 2.1. Don't worry if you do not recognise many of the drug names at this stage; the key fact here is

Table 2.1 Some common natural messengers, sub-classes of their receptors and examples of agonist and antagonist drugs that target those receptors

Natural messenger	Class of receptor	Sub-class of receptor	Key locations	Example of agonist drug	Example of antagonist drug
Adrenaline/ noradrenaline	Adrenergic	Alpha-1	Arterioles	*Phenylephrine*	*Doxazosin*
		Beta-1	Heart	*Dobutamine*	*Atenolol*
		Beta-2	Bronchioles	*Salbutamol*	None
Acetylcholine	Cholinergic	Muscarinic	Bronchioles	None	*Ipratropium*
		Nicotinic	Muscles	*Suxamethonium*	*Pancuronium*
Histamine	Histamine	H-1	Inner ear	None	*Cyclizine*
		H-2	Stomach	None	*Cimetidine*
Opioid-like peptides	Opioid	Mu	Central nervous system	*Morphine*	*Naloxone*
		Kappa		*Nalbuphine*	
		Delta		*Pentazocine*	

that the effect of the natural chemical messenger binding to its receptor depends on the sub-class and location of the receptor. Adrenaline binding to β_1 receptors on the heart increases the heart rate and force of contraction, but adrenaline binding to β_2 receptors in the bronchioles causes bronchodilation. This is very important in pharmacology because it means that drugs can be developed that target one specific sub-class of receptor. Thus a drug such as *salbutamol* is a β_2 adrenergic receptor agonist and will bind preferentially to β_2 receptors in the lungs rather than any other sub-class of adrenergic receptor. This is why we can have drugs that target specific organs or tissues such as the heart, lungs, digestive system, nervous system, etc. We also have the option of stimulating the receptor with an agonist or blocking it with an antagonist, whichever is appropriate. Table 2.1 shows that some receptors are targeted by both agonist and antagonist drugs. The key point here is that these different sub-classes of receptors provide useful pharmacological targets.

There is unfortunately a downside to the body having classes of structurally similar receptors. It is useful in that we can target a drug at a particular sub-class of receptor, expressed on a particular tissue to produce a therapeutic effect, but inevitably that drug may also bind to another member of that group and produce an unwanted effect – a side-effect. This can be a major problem with some drugs and the subject of side-effects is explored more fully in Chapter 3.

> ### KEY FACT
> Drugs can be targeted at specific sub-classes of receptors but may accidentally bind to other receptors of that class, resulting in unwanted effects (side-effects).

Drugs that bind to various classes of receptor with either agonist or antagonist actions have been given specific names that you may come across in the pharmacological literature. These terms are **sympathomimetic** and **cholinergic** (both agonist), and **anticholinergic** (antagonist).

A sympathomimetic drug such as *salbutamol* is one that mimics the action of adrenaline or noradrenaline released during sympathetic nervous activity. The bronchodilator *ipratropium* is an antagonist for acetylcholine receptors in the lungs, and therefore is anticholinergic. There are no direct agonists of acetylcholine in clinical use but *neostigmine*, a drug used to reverse muscle relaxation after surgery, is effectively cholinergic in action.

A QUICK RECAP on receptors

- Receptors are proteins found on the cell membrane and also inside cells.
- Receptors are targets for chemical messengers such as hormones, neurotransmitters and mediators.
- When a chemical messenger binds to a receptor it produces an effect in that cell.

- Drugs are of similar shape to natural chemical messengers and so bind to the same receptors.
- Agonist drugs bind to receptors and produce the same effect as the natural chemical messengers.
- Antagonist drugs bind to receptors and block them from the effects of the natural chemical messengers.
- There are sub-classes of receptors expressed on specific tissues that allow drugs to target those tissues.

2.3 Protein targets 2: ion channels

It is probable that every major physiological process in the body in some way depends on ions moving across cell membranes, either passively through ion channels or actively through carrier proteins. The rhythmic beating of the heart depends on ions moving across cell membranes, as does the swift movement of nervous impulses along the neurons of the nervous system, the absorption of nutrients by the digestive system and the filtering of waste by the kidneys. It would indeed be difficult to identify a physiological process where the movement of ions across cell membranes did not play a key part. It is hardly surprising, therefore, that the proteins that facilitate the passage of ions across cell membranes are targets of many of the drugs currently used in clinical practice.

What, therefore, are ions and why is their transport across cell membranes so crucial to the efficient functioning of the body?

Ions are atoms that carry a tiny charge (although ions can also be small molecules). Some common examples of ions found in the body are listed in Table 2.2 and, as you can see from the table, some carry a positive charge and are called **cations** and some carry a negative charge and are called **anions**. Elements such as sodium, calcium and chlorine can exist in non-ionic forms but they are unstable and very reactive and you will not find them in living organisms. The ions that we find in the body are stable and are charged. Most carry either a single positive or single negative charge – although some such as calcium, magnesium and phosphate have a double or even triple charge (hence the $^{2+}$ or $^{3-}$ in superscript after their chemical symbol).

> **KEY FACT**
> **Ions** are charged and ions are stable.

There are many other types of ion found in the human body but those listed in Table 2.2 are the ones that you are most likely to encounter in physiological processes related to pharmacology.

Table 2.2 Common ions found in the body

Name of ion	Chemical symbol	Cation or anion
Sodium	Na^+	Cation
Potassium	K^+	Cation
Calcium	Ca^{2+}	Cation
Chloride	Cl^-	Anion
Hydrogen	H^+	Cation
Magnesium	Mg^{2+}	Cation
Phosphate	$PO_4{}^{3-}$	Anion
Bicarbonate	$HCO_3{}^-$	Anion

Examples of some common drugs that interact with ion channels include:

- *Lidocaine* – local anaesthetic used in dentistry
- *Diazepam* – **anxiolytic** (relieves anxiety)
- *Digoxin* – maintains the contractility of the heart
- *Verapamil* – reduces **hypertension** (high blood pressure)

The roles that ions play in physiological processes are discussed in more detail when we examine the various body systems in Part 2 of *Introducing Pharmacology*, along with the drugs that target those systems. Here we will just look at the basic principles as to how drugs interact with ion channels.

IN PRACTICE

You will often hear the term **U & Es** used in clinical practice. It stands for **urea** and **electrolytes** and must be one of the most common blood tests performed in hospitals. The key electrolytes are Na^+ and K^+ and deviations from the normal range could indicate various problems such as dehydration. Urea, a waste product, is eliminated in the urine, so high levels in the blood may indicate that the kidneys are not functioning normally.

There are various types of ion channels that perform different tasks in different tissues but essentially they all regulate the passage of ions across the cell membrane. Some ion channels open and close as the electrical activity surrounding the membrane changes. These are called **voltage-controlled ion channels** and are found on cells involved in the transmission of **nervous impulses** such as neurons and conduction tissue in the heart (Figure 2.6).

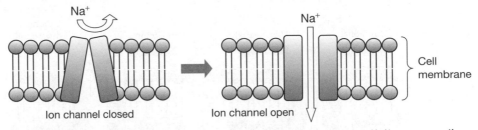

Figure 2.6 Ion channels open in response to changes in electrical activity surrounding the membrane. In this case a sodium channel opens.

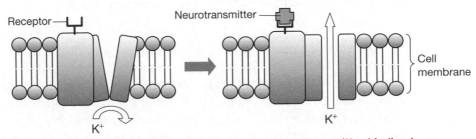

Figure 2.7 An ion channel opens in response to a neurotransmitter binding to an associated receptor protein. In this case a potassium channel opens.

Some ion channels are complexed with receptors. These are found in various locations but especially at the junctions between neurons. As the neurotransmitter released by one neuron binds to a receptor on another neuron, this causes the associated ion channel to open (Figure 2.7).

So how do drugs interact with ion channels? Some drugs simply block the ion channel by inserting themselves into the channel itself and preventing the passage of ions from one side of the membrane to the other. An example of a drug that has this action is the local anaesthetic *lidocaine*.

Example of a channel-blocking drug: *lidocaine*

Lidocaine is a synthetic relation of cocaine and is commonly used as a local anaesthetic to prevent patients experiencing pain during minor operations such as dentistry. As you lie back in the dentist's chair for a filling and the dentist approaches with a syringe, the last thought in your mind is probably about the way that *lidocaine* will make the whole process relatively pain free. However, without *lidocaine*, fillings would be a lot more painful, so read on to find out how this most useful of drugs works.

Figure 2.8 shows a section of the cell membrane of a pain neuron that transmits unpleasant sensations from the site of damage into the central nervous system. Pain impulses, in fact all nervous impulses, depend on Na^+ ions entering the neuron through voltage-controlled sodium ion channels. Changes in the electrical activity around the neuron membrane stimulate sodium channels to open, and

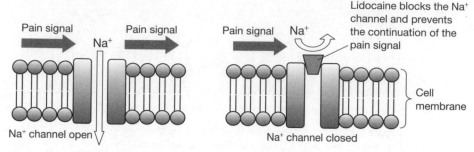

Figure 2.8 Blocking the sodium channels in a pain neuron with *lidocaine* prevents pain signals from progressing along the neuron and reaching the brain.

Na^+ ions enter the neuron causing a change in the electrical activity around the membrane that causes adjacent sodium channels to open – and so on along the neuron. This is the nervous impulse, or **action potential** as it is more correctly called, sending a ripple of ionic activity along the neuron, rather like a Mexican wave at a football match. Naturally there is more to it than this brief explanation and other ions such as potassium are involved, but for this brief example of a channel-blocking drug, you just need to know that pain impulses depend on the opening of sodium channels in pain neurons.

Lidocaine and other related local anaesthetics are blockers of sodium channels in pain neurons. They bind to, and block, the sodium channel so that sodium ions cannot enter the neuron and this prevents the progression of the nervous impulse along the pain neuron. Since the perception of pain depends on the brain receiving pain signals from pain neurons, local anaesthetics effectively sever communications between the site of injury and the brain. *Lidocaine* will act preferentially on pain neurons but can also affect the motor neurons that control muscles and prevent their proper functioning – as anyone who has had a dental filling and afterwards tried to speak normally will confirm.

Other drugs affect ion channels differently and these are called **modulators**. Two such examples are the anti-anxiety drug *diazepam* and the antihypertensive drug *verapamil*. Modulators change the way that ion channels behave, either enhancing or inhibiting their action. *Diazepam* interacts with chloride channels in neurons of the central nervous system and enhances their opening, so encouraging the movement of chloride ions out of the neuron. *Verapamil* inhibits the opening of calcium channels in the heart and prevents Ca^{2+} entering heart cells, which has the effect of slowing the heart. How these drugs achieve this modulation is quite complex and perhaps best left for a more advanced level study of pharmacology.

> In my BNF, verapamil is listed as a calcium channel blocker – no mention of a modulator.

Well spotted, but even though *verapamil* is listed in the BNF as a calcium channel blocker (CCB), it does not in fact block calcium channels in the same way that *lidocaine* blocks sodium channels. The word 'modulate' just means to change, so if the BNF uses the popular term *blocker*, it is still a meaningful description of *verapamil*'s action.

2.4 Protein targets 3: enzymes

Within each cell there are thousands of tiny biochemical reactions taking place every second, mostly involving enzymes, large, complex proteins that **catalyse** those reactions. These reactions are not easy to describe in simple terms without delving deeper into biochemistry but, basically, enzymes change one substance into another substance – for instance, by removing (or adding) a phosphate, breaking (or making) a bond between two carbon atoms and so on. Each enzyme is responsible for catalysing one particular type of biochemical reaction, which it can do time and time again because the enzyme itself remains unchanged by the reaction. The substance that an enzyme converts into another substance is called the **substrate** of that enzyme.

> To **catalyse** a chemical reaction is to speed up the rate of that reaction by a **catalyst** (such as an enzyme). However, the catalyst itself is not changed by that reaction.

There are many thousands of different enzymes active inside and outside of cells, and they are responsible for the catalysis of the myriad biochemical reactions necessary for life. Few of them have memorable names, in fact some of them have abominably long names that few of us can pronounce, let alone remember. Table 2.3 shows some of the enzymes that we will need to know because they are targets for drugs.

How do drugs interact with enzymes?

Drugs generally inhibit enzymes and prevent them from performing their normal physiological tasks. This inhibition is caused by drugs binding to the **active site** of the enzyme, the area where the enzyme interacts with its substrate. Drugs that inhibit enzymes have a molecular shape similar to the substrate; they bind to the active site and inhibit the action of the enzyme (Figure 2.9).

Table 2.3 Some enzyme targets and the drugs that target them

Enzyme target	Drug group	Use
Angiotensin-converting enzyme	ACE inhibitors	Antihypertensive
Cyclo-oxygenase II	NSAIDs*	Analgesic
HMG CoA reductase†	Statins	Reduces cholesterol
Topoisomerase II	Cytotoxic antibiotics	Leukaemia and lymphoma

* Non-steroidal anti-inflammatory drugs
† 3-hydroxy-3-methylglutaryl coenzyme A reductase (phew . . . !!!)

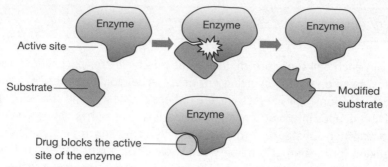

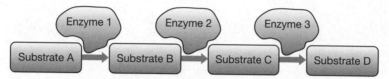

Figure 2.9 The active site in an enzyme modifies a substrate. A drug with similarities in shape to the substrate occupies the active site and prevents the enzyme from binding to its substrate.

Figure 2.10 A biochemical pathway where substrate A is converted into substrate D via a series of intermediate steps, each catalysed by its own enzyme.

Many enzyme-blocking drugs are targeted at enzymes in **biochemical pathways** and it is important to know what this term means. In cells, substances are synthesised, not in one complex manoeuvre, but in a series of small stages, each change being carried out by a different enzyme (Figure 2.10).

ANOTHER WAY TO PICTURE THIS

Rather like the assembly line in a car factory, each worker (enzyme) has his own small task to perform, adding components such as the engine, exhaust, wheels and windows until at the end of the line a finished car is produced.

In Figure 2.11, a drug has blocked the action of enzyme 2. As a result, the pathway is blocked and neither substrate C nor D is produced. It is invariably the final substance in the biochemical pathway that we are trying to prevent being produced. For example, statins such as *pravastatin* and *atorvastatin* block an enzyme in the pathway that produces cholesterol in the liver. High cholesterol in the blood is a contributory factor to coronary artery disease, so reducing

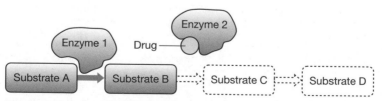

Figure 2.11 A drug binding to the active site of enzyme 2 blocks the pathway by preventing the conversion of substrate B into substrate C.

cholesterol synthesis with a statin helps to prevent heart attacks. The action of statins is discussed in more detail in Chapter 4.

2.5 Protein targets 4: carrier proteins

Of all of the protein drug targets, the carrier proteins form the least coherent group, comprising any membrane protein involved in the active transport of a substance across the cell membrane using ATP as the motive force. For the sake of simplicity we can divide carrier proteins into two broad categories.

The first group of carrier proteins, confusingly perhaps, are those that transport ions across membranes. We have already encountered voltage-controlled ion channels relying on simple diffusion, but some ions are actively transported or pumped across membranes through carrier proteins using ATP. Figure 2.12 shows an ATP-driven carrier protein.

These ion pumps are found on cell membranes in various parts of the body, but those in the kidneys and lining of the stomach are among the most common targets for drugs. *Furosemide*, a **loop diuretic**, inhibits an ion carrier in the **loop of Henle**, part of the **nephrons** of the kidney. This interferes with the sodium balance in the kidney, causing it to increase its production of urine. For patients with **heart failure**, removing fluid from the body can reduce the workload of the heart.

> **Nephrons** are the tiny filtration tubes found by the million in each kidney. They are responsible for controlling the production of urine and the removal of wastes from the blood.

Lansoprazole, a **proton pump inhibitor** (PPI), inhibits the hydrogen ion (proton) pump in the gastric mucosa of the stomach. The pumping of hydrogen ions increases the concentration of **hydrochloric acid** in the stomach which, in some patients, can cause irritation of the lower **oesophagus**, a problem known as **gastro-oesophageal reflux** (heartburn). Blocking the proton pump with a PPI results in a reduction in the amount of stomach acid which helps to alleviate the symptoms.

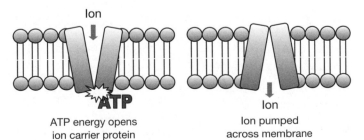

Ion

ATP

ATP energy opens
ion carrier protein

Ion

Ion pumped
across membrane

Figure 2.12 ATP-driven carrier protein moves an ion across a membrane.

The second group of carrier proteins targeted by drugs are those found in the junctions between neurons in the complex neural circuits in the brain. These drugs are used in mental health to relieve depression and are dealt with in more detail in Chapter 11. *Fluoxetine* and *paroxetine*, perhaps better known by their trade names of Prozac® and Seroxat®, are anxiolytic drugs that block the 5-hydroxytryptamine (serotonin) carrier proteins in neurons in the emotional centres of the brain. How this results in positive changes in mood is complex and by no means fully understood.

A QUICK RECAP on ion channels, enzymes and carrier proteins

- Ion channels in the cell membrane allow ions to enter and leave the cell.

- Most physiological processes involve the movement of ions across membranes, especially nervous conduction and heart activity.

- Some drugs simply block ion channels. Other drugs modulate them which enhances or inhibits the passage of ions across membranes.

- Enzymes are large, complex proteins that act as catalysts in biochemical reactions.

- Enzyme-blocking drugs inhibit the action of enzymes and prevent them binding to their substrate. This often inhibits biochemical pathways.

- Carrier proteins move ions and various other molecules across membranes using ATP as an energy source.

- Drugs acting on carrier proteins generally block the carrier but the effect varies with the type and location of carrier.

RUNNING WORDS

Here are some of the technical terms that were included in this chapter.
Read them one by one and tick them off when you are sure that you understand them.

5-Hydroxytryptamine p. 40
Acetylcholine p. 26
Action potential p. 36
Active site p. 37
Adrenaline p. 26
Adrenergic p. 31
Adrenoceptor p. 31
Agonist p. 29
Anion p. 33
Antagonist p. 29
Anti-cholinergic p. 32
Anxiolytic p. 34
Arteriole p. 26
Beta-1 adrenaline receptors p. 31
Beta-2 adrenaline receptors p. 31

Biochemical pathway p. 38
Blockers p. 29
Catalyse p. 37
Catalysts p. 37
Cation p. 33
Cholinergic p. 32
Electrolyte p. 34
Endogenous ligand p. 27
Gastro-oesophageal reflux p. 39
Heart failure p. 39
Histamine p. 26
Homeostasis p. 25
Hormone p. 26
Hydrochloric acid p. 39
Hypertension p. 34
Insulin p. 26
Loop diuretic p. 39

Loop of Henle p. 39
Mediator p. 26
Modulator p. 36
Nephrons p. 39
Nervous impulses p. 34
Neurotransmitter p. 26
Noradrenaline p. 26
Oesophagus p. 39
Parasympathetic p. 26
Proton pump inhibitor p. 39
Serotonin p. 40
Specificity p. 27
Substrate p. 37
Sympathetic p. 26
Sympathomimetic p. 32
Urea p. 34
Voltage-controlled ion channel p. 34

REFERENCES AND FURTHER RECOMMENDED READING

Rang, H.P. *et al.* (2007) *Rang and Dale's Pharmacology* (6th edition). Churchill Livingstone. Section 1 provides an in-depth examination of the principles of molecular drug action.

Your turn to try

Now you have finished reading this chapter it's time to find out how much you have learned and remembered. Don't worry if you can't answer all of the questions and have to reread parts of Chapter 2 – this is all part of the learning process.

The answers to these questions are at the end of the book on page 283.

1 Approximately how many different proteins are there in the human body?

2 Outline three reasons that proteins make good targets for drugs.

3 Name three types of natural chemical messenger that target receptors.

4 How do natural chemical messengers target their receptors?

5 Why does salbutamol bind to adrenergic receptors?

6 Explain the terms *agonist* and *antagonist*.

7 Explain the term *sympathomimetic*.

8 What type of natural chemical messenger would bind to nicotinic and muscarinic receptors?

9 Cations are *negatively / positively* charged ions (delete incorrect option)

10 What type of ion channels open in response to changes in electrical activity across the cell membrane?

11 What is the effect of *lidocaine* blocking Na^+ channels in pain neurons?

12 Which part of an enzyme is blocked by enzyme-blocking drugs?

13 What biochemical pathway do statins inhibit?

14 What is the key difference between an ion channel and a carrier protein?

Answers to questions on page 22

1 Phospholipids and cholesterol.
2 Protein synthesis.
3 Amino acids.
4 A gene.
5 Oxygen
6 Glycogen.

Answers to match the lock and key in Figure 2.3, page 28

Lock 1 – key C
Lock 2 – key A
Lock 3 – key B

Chapter 3

Side-effects, interactions and pharmacokinetics

AIMS

By the time you have finished the chapter you will:

1 Understand the principles of pharmacokinetics – how absorption, metabolism and elimination affects drug levels in the body.
2 Understand how factors such as disease and age can affect metabolism and elimination.
3 Understand the different ways that drugs may cause side-effects.
4 Understand how some drugs may interact with other drugs (and some foods).
5 Understand factors that determine the correct dosage of drugs.

CONTENTS

Introduction

In Chapter 1 we examined the structure and function of cells and looked at some basic biochemistry. In Chapter 2 we examined the four key protein targets for drugs - receptors, ion channels, enzymes and carrier proteins, and we also looked at a few examples of the drugs that interacted with these protein targets. These first two chapters are very important because they will enable you to understand how the drug interacts with the body to produce its therapeutic effect. This is the subject of the second part of this book where we look at the major drug groups and how they interact with cells and tissues, mainly by binding to our four groups of target proteins.

In this chapter we are going to take a step sideways to explore the subject of pharmacokinetics. Rather than explaining the therapeutic effects of the drug on the body, pharmacokinetics is concerned with what the body does to the drug, how drugs are absorbed into the body, metabolised (usually by the liver) and eventually eliminated. It is an important topic because it explains why some drugs must be delivered directly into the bloodstream while others can be taken orally, in tablet or liquid form. It also explains why some drugs can be given once a day while others need to be administered more frequently. Disease and age can have a profound effect on drug metabolism, which is another area we will touch on briefly.

The next part of Chapter 3 examines the important and problematical area of side-effects. It may seem slightly odd that after only two chapters and before we have even started to discuss the therapeutic action of drugs, we are about to examine how they cause side-effects. If we lived in an ideal world, then we might indeed be able to design drugs that cured diseases and never caused any other problems. In reality, however, we are dealing with the human body which is an extremely complex machine and, inevitably, introducing foreign chemicals into that complex machine has the potential to interfere with its normal, efficient running. If you have a *British National Formulary* nearby, open it at any page, choose any drug and check whether it has the potential to cause side-effects. You may (or may not) be surprised to find that every single drug in the BNF has one or more entries under the heading of 'side-effects' - some have dozens of entries. This does not, of course, mean that everyone who is prescribed a particular drug will experience these side-effects but it is important for you as a clinical practitioner, who may be involved in the administration of that drug, to be aware of the potential for it to cause problems. You not only need to be aware of the potential side-effects of a drug but also the mechanism whereby it can produce those side-effects. This knowledge will enable you to anticipate potential problems, identify them and respond to them quickly - before they become more serious. In Part 2 of *Introducing Pharmacology*, we shall be examining not only the therapeutic actions of key groups of drugs but also how they produce side-effects, so by introducing this subject in Part 1, you will be well prepared for this aspect of pharmacology.

Chapter 3 continues with an exploration of another important area – interactions. Many of your patients will have multiple pathologies and will have been prescribed more than one drug. In this case there is the potential for the drugs to interact, meaning that one drug may change the activity of another. It may increase the other drug's activity to the point where it starts to become toxic or it may reduce that drug's activity to the point where it ceases to have any therapeutic benefit. Both of these situations can be potentially serious – even fatal. Strangely, it is not just drugs that can interact with each other. Common foods such as grapefruit and cabbage can change the activity of some drugs – as can common herbal remedies available off the shelf in health-food shops. The problems of interactions are compounded in patients with **chronic** (long-term) disease who are often on a cocktail of drugs, greatly increasing the potential for interactions. It is important therefore that you understand the principles of interactions and be wary when administering drugs to these patients. Remember that the person who administers a drug has a responsibility for the safe use of that drug – not just the person who prescribes it.

Finally in Chapter 3 we examine the factors that determine the dose of a drug that should be administered to a patient. If an insufficient amount is administered, it may not produce the desired therapeutic effect. Conversely, if too much is given, it may produce unacceptable levels of side-effects and even harm the patient. Giving patients the correct dose ensures that the level of drug in the body is appropriate and helps to prevent these potential problems.

WHERE ARE WE STARTING FROM?

This is the third chapter of *Introducing Pharmacology* so you should be starting to get familiar with life at a cellular and even biochemical level where most drugs work. Let's start off with a short quiz to check how much you have remembered from Chapters 1 and 2.

1 Amino acids are the main components of what class of biological molecules?

_____

2 What is the role of ATP in cells?

_____

3 Triglycerides are what type of biological molecule?

_____

4 Name three classes of chemical messengers that bind to receptors.

_____

5 Receptor-blocking drugs are called . . . ?

_____

Answers are at the end of the chapter on page 69.

How did you do? If you got most of the answers correct then you have under-stood and remembered most of the previous two chapters. If you only got one or two answers correct, then it might be useful to reread the first two chapters because a lot of the terms that we encountered there will reappear in this chapter – and indeed the rest of the book. Few of us remember or understand everything at the first reading, so don't worry if you need to read each section a few times before it makes sense.

3.1 Pharmacokinetics: what the body does to drugs

Up to this point in *Introducing Pharmacology* we have been mainly concerned with what drugs do to the body. Now we are going to look at what the body does to drugs.

Have you ever wondered why is it that some drugs are administered orally, perhaps in tablet form, while others can only be given by injection? Why is it that some drugs are given once each day, others three times each day while others need continuous administration? The answer to these questions lies in the way that the body absorbs, **metabolises** and eliminates the drugs that we administer to patients.

> **Metabolise** simply means to change by a biochemical reaction. Much of the metabolic activity relating to drugs takes place in the liver.

We must remember that the body is blind to the nature of foreign substances such as drugs – it does not know that these beneficial chemicals have been administered to treat or prevent a disease. To the body, drugs are foreign substances and, like all foreign substances, the body will place barriers to prevent their entry, neutralise those that do gain entry and then dispose of them as quickly as possible. Drug manufacturers have to take these reactions into account when developing a new drug. It is obviously important to ensure that the drug is effective against the dis-ease for which it is being prescribed, but it must also survive the barriers to entry and subsequent neutralisation by the liver. It must also stay in the circulation long enough to do its job as a therapeutic agent but not so long that it continues to act long after its usefulness to the patient has ended. It is therefore important to understand the principles of pharmacokinetics in order to understand the reason for the route of delivery, the frequency of administration and also to appreciate that factors such as age and disease can affect how the drug will act in the body.

We can divide the way that the body deals with drugs into three stages . . .

- The absorption of drugs into the body
- The metabolism of drugs by the body
- The elimination of drugs from the body.

The absorption of drugs into the body

To act effectively, drugs need to find their way to the site of the disease. We can broadly divide the routes of administration into three major categories:

1 **Topical** – the medication is applied directly to the site of the problem where the drug needs to act. This is often (but not always) the skin.

2 **Enteral** – the medication is taken orally and absorbed into the blood stream from the digestive tract. (Note that some drugs may need to remain in the digestive tract if they are to treat digestive tract diseases.)

3 **Parenteral** – the medication is introduced directly into the body usually by **intramuscular** injection (into a muscle) or **intravenously** (into a vein).

A pictorial summary of the various routes of administration is given in Figure 3.1.

Topical administration Sometimes the problem is localised so near the surface of the body that the drug can be applied directly to the skin. ***Hydrocortisone***, a topical corticosteroid used for eczema, is an example of a drug applied directly to the skin. Some inhaled drugs such as ***salbutamol*** and ***ipratropium bromide*** probably fit best in this category as they are delivered into and act on the lung tissue.

Enteral administration The oral administration of drugs is perhaps the most acceptable method to the conscious and cooperative patient because, given the choice, most people prefer to take a couple of tablets than have a hypodermic needle stuck into them! Drugs taken orally must be sufficiently robust to withstand the rigours of the digestive system such as stomach acid and digestive enzymes. If the drug has survived its passage through the stomach and duodenum into the **jejunum** (middle, absorptive section of the small intestine), it will start to be absorbed into the circulatory system and here we encounter the first of the body's

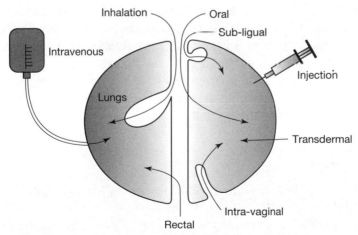

Figure 3.1 There are many ways to introduce drugs into the body. The route chosen depends on various factors, including the nature of the drug, the pathology, the state of the patient and the required response time.

defences against foreign substances – the liver. This organ plays a major role in drug metabolism and we will shortly discuss it in more detail.

Parenteral administration   This really covers any drug that is not administered orally, and while the term is generally applied to injections and **intravenous** (IV) lines, it can also cover other routes. Injection is an effective way of introducing a drug quickly into a **subcutaneous** (under the skin) area. Sometimes the drug stays in the area of injection such as the dental anaesthetic *lidocaine.* Other drugs such as *insulin* diffuse from the site of injection into the bloodstream for distribution around the body. *Insulin* is an example of a drug that cannot survive the passage through the digestive tract. As a protein, it would be quickly denatured by digestive enzymes and unlikely to reach the bloodstream. Drugs administered directly into a vein or artery have an almost immediate effect as there is little of the transport delay that occurs between the gut and the blood as in the case of oral administration. This type of delivery is very suitable where the amount of drug in the blood stream must be carefully controlled. For example, *morphine* used to control severe pain is often delivered IV by a dispenser controlled by the patient. As the pain levels increase, the patient is able to obtain almost immediate relief by increasing the rate of delivery of the *morphine*. This is called **patient-controlled analgesia** – or PCA for short.

There are some drugs that fall between categories. These are drugs that have a systemic action but are not delivered orally or by injection or IV. These are drugs that pass through one of the body's membranes to be absorbed into the blood stream. Various membranes can be used to absorb drugs, for example the **sub-lingual** (under-the-tongue) route can be useful for drugs that cannot survive the trip through the stomach to the blood stream such as the anti-angina drug *glyceryl trinitrate*. Rectal delivery by incorporating the drug into **suppositories** can be useful for those unable to take medication by mouth, for example analgesia for patients who are recovering from an operation. The absorption of drugs **transdermally** (through the skin) is generally poor but highly lipid soluble drugs such as anti-inflammatory **corticosteroids** and the hormone **oestrogen** can be delivered successfully by this route. Drugs delivered via the lungs are quite common, such as the general anaesthetics *sevoflurane* and *nitrous oxide* that quickly pass into the bloodstream and thence to the brain.

IN PRACTICE

It is very important that drugs are administered by the correct route because often the doses can vary between routes. Generally IV doses are much smaller than enteral doses because of drug metabolism in the liver situated between the gut and the circulatory system. There have been several cases of fatalities where drugs have been delivered by the wrong route.

The metabolism of drugs by the body

Once the drug has survived its passage through the stomach and into the duodenum and jejunum of the small intestine, it will start to be absorbed into the circulatory system. Here we encounter the first of the body's defences against foreign substances – the liver.

Firstly, we need to learn a bit of anatomy relating to the circulatory and digestive system. Most tissues and organs have conventional plumbing consisting of an artery that supplies them with oxygenated blood and a vein that removes the deoxygenated blood and returns it to the general circulation. The digestive system, however, has a slight variation on this theme for although it has a conventional blood supply via the **mesenteric artery**, the blood is returned by a vein that feeds directly into the liver – rather than into the general circulation. This vein is called the **hepatic portal vein** and ensures that all of the nutrients and other substances that we absorb from the gut first pass through the liver (Figure 3.2).

Why do the all the nutrients and miscellaneous substances absorbed from the digestive system have to first pass through the liver? Well, imagine you have just been out for a birthday meal with your pals and as a special treat you have a double helping of sticky toffee pudding and custard (it is your birthday after all). Very nice indeed, but imagine the effect on your blood glucose levels if all the

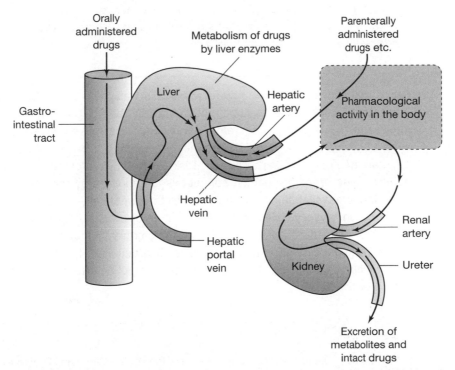

Figure 3.2 Summary of drug metabolism in the body. Drugs in the digestive system travel through the liver before being released into the general circulatory system.

sugar from that pudding emptied directly into your circulation from your intestine! Fortunately, the sugars firstly feed into the liver via the hepatic portal vein where most of them are stored as glycogen. This means that the blood leaving the liver via the **hepatic vein** will not be excessively high in sugars compared to normal blood.

The liver not only acts as a **buffer** to nutrients absorbed from the digestive system, it also acts as a barrier to unwanted substances and potential toxins. These substances appear naturally in our food and include numerous chemicals from plants and animal products, most of which are not particularly toxic but still need to be processed before they enter the bloodstream. The liver also acts as the body's main 'detox' organ, breaking down and neutralising substances that have been produced in metabolic reactions in the cells and tissues. These include hormones and other substances that have fulfilled their purpose and need to be removed from the system.

The mechanism whereby the liver performs this valuable task involves a family of metabolising enzymes called **cytochrome P450 (microsomal)** enzymes, different families specialising in breaking down different substances. Among the substances that the P450 enzymes break down are drugs, and this has important implications for drug delivery and, as we shall see later in this chapter, drug interactions.

> A **buffer** is a structure, substance or process that resists or helps to prevent change. In this case, the liver acts to prevent major changes in blood nutrients after a meal.

Drugs that are absorbed from the digestive tract all pass through the liver and to a greater or lesser extent will be metabolised by the P450 enzymes before they enter into the circulatory system. This is called **first-pass metabolism** and the extent of the metabolism will determine the amount of a drug that appears in the circulation to perform its therapeutic task – sometimes referred to as its **bioavailability**. Some drugs are almost completely metabolised by the liver, resulting in such low bioavailability that the drug is therapeutically ineffective. The anti-angina drug *glyceryl trinitrate* is an example of a drug subject to almost complete first-pass metabolism, which is why it is generally delivered by sub-lingual spray. From under the tongue, GTN will be absorbed directly into the bloodstream and will have just enough time to exert its therapeutic effect before being inactivated by the liver.

> **KEY FACT**
> **P450 enzymes** in the liver play a key role in drug metabolism. They metabolise both drugs absorbed from the digestive tract and those already in the system.

If you return to Figure 3.2 above, you will see that parenteral drugs, introduced directly into the circulation by IV line, etc., will also pass through the liver where they come into contact with P450 metabolising enzymes. As the blood circulates around the body, drugs carried in the blood are subject to hepatic metabolism each time they pass through the liver. How long a drug remains in the circulation depends on various factors, including how quickly it is metabolised by the P450 enzymes. However, enough of the drug needs to remain in the circulation to diffuse from the blood into the tissues and perform its therapeutic task. Interestingly, some drugs are inactive until metabolised by the liver. These are called **pro-drugs** and include *enalapril* (an anti-hypertensive ACE inhibitor) and the anti-clotting drugs *aspirin* and *clopidogrel*.

> **Bioavailability** is a commonly used but rather imprecise term that refers to the amount of drug, generally in the circulation, available to perform its therapeutic activity.

The elimination of drugs from the body

As we have just discussed, most drugs are metabolised by the liver into **metabolites**. This often involves adding a sugar molecule to the drug in order that it will become more soluble in blood which makes it easier for the kidneys to remove it from the body. The kidneys are the main excretion organs of the body, acting as complex filter beds; they remove unwanted materials from the blood while conserving the useful materials such as glucose, salts and amino acids. In this manner drugs and their metabolites eventually find their way to the kidneys where they are filtered out of the blood and appear in the urine. A few drugs are eliminated by the liver in the **bile**, a mixture of cholesterol, acids and pigments that is transported to the digestive system via the bile duct. This empties into the duodenum and plays an important part in fat digestion.

> **DID YOU KNOW . . .** that urine tests in sport are searching for tell-tale traces of metabolites that indicate the athlete concerned has been using performance-enhancing drugs? Some athletes try to evade detection by using substances naturally produced in the body such as testosterone and **erythropoietin**, but testing is now able to detect illegal usage and use that information to catch the drug cheats.

Any problem affecting the kidney has the potential to change the rate of elimination and this can affect the amount of a particular drug in the circulation. As well as kidney disease, normal ageing processes can reduce the rate of renal clearance in the elderly and so increase the bioavailability of drugs. With age, the liver also tends to become less efficient, which means that drugs are broken down more slowly, again increasing their bioavailability. This reduction in liver efficiency can also affect first-pass metabolism, allowing more of the drug absorbed from the gut to reach the circulatory system. These factors mean that one needs to be very careful when administering drugs to elderly people, especially those drugs where an increase in circulating levels could cause problematic side-effects.

Newly born babies also need special consideration because their liver and kidneys are not fully developed and metabolism and elimination is less efficient. However, there are very few drugs licensed for such young children and prescribing for them is limited to those with experience in paediatric medicine.

IN PRACTICE

Any disease that affects the liver or kidneys can have an effect on the bioavailability of drugs. Cirrhosis of the liver reduces its ability to metabolise drugs, which means that circulating drug levels are elevated. Renal failure means that drugs are excreted more slowly, again elevating levels in the circulation.

3.2 How drugs can cause side-effects

There is a popular saying in pharmacology that goes . . .

'A drug that does not cause side-effects is a drug that does not work.'

No one is quite sure who first said this but, unlike most popular sayings, this one is invariably true. All drugs have the potential to cause **side-effects** and a quick glance at the BNF will confirm this. Some drugs may cause relatively few side-effects while the list of side-effects for other drugs is so long that one wonders why anyone would ever prescribe them.

Why would we use these drugs if we know that they may cause side-effects?

Firstly, some patients will experience few, if any, side-effects and if those side-effects are relatively minor then the therapeutic benefit of a drug will generally outweigh any problems. For example, a slight feeling of nausea may be acceptable if an antibacterial drug rids us of a painful throat infection.

Secondly, the condition of the patient may be so serious that even quite unpleasant side-effects may be tolerated if it ensures the patient's recovery. For example, drugs used to treat cancer can have very unpleasant side-effects but if they save the individual's life, then that will be a price worth paying.

So why do patients experience different side-effects?

This is a good question but unfortunately not an easy one to answer. Basically, everyone is physically different and these differences can be observed in people's height, weight, hair colour, facial features, body shape, etc. There are also differences within the body, in particular in the way that our bodies deal with drugs. Most of these differences manifest themselves at a cellular level which is where drugs interact with the body. Drugs target specific proteins and these proteins can differ between individuals, which means that our response to drugs can differ – both in their therapeutic effect and in their ability to cause side-effects. The way that our bodies absorb, metabolise and eliminate drugs differs between individuals, perhaps because of age or disease, and this can result in variations in the amount of drug circulating in the blood. This can affect both the therapeutic and unwanted effects – as we will see later in this chapter.

Drugs also differ in their tendency to cause side-effects. Some drugs cause many side-effects whereas others cause fewer problems. Some drugs regularly cause minor inconveniences such as nausea but rarely cause any serious problems. Other drugs quite regularly cause unpleasant side-effects and need monitoring carefully. The message is that every drug is different and it will behave differently in each individual patient. This is not, of course, to imply that there is a complete lack of predictability with the drugs that we administer but, because of individual differences, there will inevitably be some variation between patients both with regard to their therapeutic response and their susceptibility to side-effects.

> **KEY FACT**
> Patients will differ in their response to drugs, especially with the **side-effects** they may experience.

How drugs can cause side-effects 1: tipping the balance too far

Individuals react differently to drugs and their response can vary with factors such as age, disease and simply the normal genetic variability between people. Manufacturers are aware of this and during the testing process they decide the appropriate dosage that will provide the optimum therapeutic effect with the minimum of side-effects. However, sometimes the factors that produce a variable response to a drug are such that the drug delivers a more pronounced therapeutic effect than originally intended. Now you might think that this is a good thing because a patient who experiences an enhanced therapeutic effect will automatically be better off. This however, is not always the case. If the drug is attempting to return a physiological factor such as high blood pressure to normal, a super-efficient drug action can actually tip the patient too far to the other side of normal – into **hypotension** (low blood pressure).

ANOTHER WAY TO PICTURE THIS

Think of your central heating system at home that is controlled by a thermostat that allows you to set the temperature of your house. If the house is too cold you turn the thermostat up, but if you turn it too far, an hour later you are boiling. This is like a drug that has a greater effect than intended and tips the balance the other way.

Other examples include the anti-clotting drugs *warfarin* and *heparin* that can tip the balance of blood **coagulation** too far in the other direction and cause **haemorrhage** (unwanted bleeding). Stimulant laxatives such as *senna* can prove to be too effective and cause diarrhoea, and *codeine phosphate* used in acute diarrhoea can work too well and cause constipation.

Most examples of drugs tipping the balance too far are dependent on the dose, therefore we say that the effect is **dose related**. The greater the dose, the more pronounced is the action of the drug and the greater is the side-effect produced.

How drugs can cause side-effects 2: hitting the wrong target

We learned in Chapters 1 and 2 that most drugs bind to protein targets such as receptors, enzymes, ion channels and carrier proteins and they bind because their shape is compatible with specific regions of those proteins. In the case of drugs that bind to receptors, they are of a similar shape to the natural chemical messengers of the body and so bind to the messengers' target receptors – either stimulating or blocking those receptors. We compared this action to a key fitting into a lock, the drug being similar to the key and the receptor to the lock.

We also learned in Chapter 2 that there are sub-classes of receptor to the natural chemical messengers. For example, there are two sub-classes of adrenergic (adrenaline and noradrenaline) receptor, designated by the Greek letters alpha (α) and beta (β). These two sub-classes are further divided into α_1, α_2 and β_1, β_2. Different tissues may have different sub-classes of receptor, for example β_1 receptors are found on the heart and β_2 receptors occur in the lungs. Adrenaline binding to β_1 receptors on the heart causes **tachycardia** (an increase in heart rate), whereas adrenaline binding to β_2 receptors on the bronchioles of the lungs causes **bronchodilation** (widening of the airways) – Figure 3.3.

REALITY CHECK

Are you sure that you understand the principle that different tissues display different sub-classes of receptor to the same hormone, e.g. adrenaline? Do you understand that adrenaline binding to the various sub-classes of receptor results in different effects in those tissues?

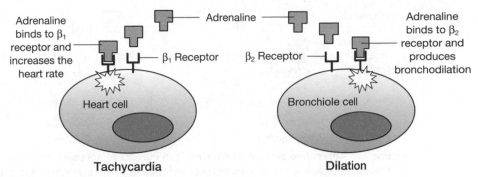

Figure 3.3 Adrenaline binding to different sub-classes of adrenergic receptor produces diverse effects in different tissues.

Table 3.1 The effects of adrenaline binding to various adrenergic receptors

Sub-class of receptor	Key locations	Effect of adrenaline binding to receptor	Physiological effect
Alpha-1 (α_1)	Arterioles	Vasoconstriction	Redirects blood from skin and maintains blood pressure
Beta-1 (β_1)	Heart	Tachycardia	Increases cardiac output
Beta-2 (β_2)	Bronchioles	Bronchodilation	Increases gas exchange in the lungs
Beta-2 (β_2)	Arteries	Vasodilation	Redirects blood to exercising muscles

This is an example of impressive economy in the body. By releasing just one hormone, adrenaline, during danger or stress, a variety of responses can be generated, appropriate to the situation – bronchodilation, tachycardia, **vasodilation** in some arteries and **vasoconstriction** in others. These different responses are possible because when adrenaline binds to the various adrenergic receptors it produces diverse effects in the tissues, dependent on the sub-class of receptor expressed on those tissues – Table 3.1.

The most striking illustration of this principle is that adrenaline binding to adrenaline receptors can cause both vasodilation and vasoconstriction. In the small **smooth muscle cells** that lie in bands around the peripheral arterioles in the skin, adrenaline binds to α_1 receptors and results in contraction of those muscle cells and thus vasoconstriction. This helps to maintain blood pressure and also to redirect blood to essential organs and muscles. Meanwhile, adrenaline binding to β_2 receptors on the muscle cells of the arteries that supply the skeletal muscles causes relaxation and vasodilation, which brings oxygen-rich blood to those muscles (Figure 3.4).

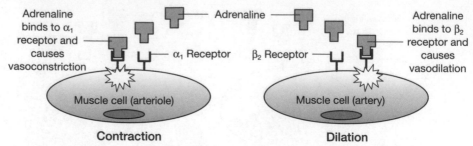

Figure 3.4 Adrenaline binding to different sub-classes of adrenergic receptor on smooth muscle cells produces vasoconstriction in peripheral arterioles and vasodilation in arteries that supply muscles.

ANOTHER WAY TO PICTURE THIS

Think of the key to your car as a hormone. It can produce two different effects depending on which lock (receptor) it goes into. The key will fit into your car door lock and open the door and also fit into your ignition lock and start your engine. One key, two locks and two different effects.

Example of side-effects 1: *salbutamol* and tachycardia

In Chapter 2 we briefly considered the anti-asthma drug *salbutamol* as an example of a drug that targets β_2 adrenergic receptors in the bronchioles of the lungs and causes bronchodilation. The molecular structure of *salbutamol* is similar to that of adrenaline and so also binds to adrenaline receptors – and produces the same effect as adrenaline, i.e. bronchodilation. As *salbutamol* is a drug that mimics adrenaline – a sympathetic system hormone – it is called a **sympathomimetic.** As it binds to and stimulates its target receptor, it is called an agonist. We will continue using this drug as an example, but will now consider how it can cause unwanted effects.

According to the *British National Formulary*, *salbutamol* can cause a variety of side-effects such as fine **tremor** (shaking), muscle cramps, **palpitations** (heart flutter) and tachycardia (fast heart rate). As mentioned earlier, some patients will experience none of these side-effects while others may experience several of them. Why should a drug that targets the bronchioles in the lungs produce so many unwanted effects on other diverse tissues and organs in the body? A few minutes thought will give us the answer. We know that *salbutamol* is a drug that mimics the action of adrenaline because it is similar in shape to adrenaline. We also know that adrenaline binds to different sub-classes of adrenergic receptor on various organs and tissues and produces a variety of effects. Logically therefore, *salbutamol* as an adrenaline agonist must also be binding to those different sub-classes of adrenergic receptors and so producing unwanted effects.

KEY FACT

Many **side-effects** are caused by drugs binding to unintended targets and producing unwanted effects.

Let us take the side-effect of tachycardia as an example. We already know that adrenaline binds to β_1 adrenergic receptors on the heart and increases the heart rate, so it is not surprising that *salbutamol*, a drug that mimics adrenaline, can also bind to β_1 receptors and speed up the heart (Figure 3.5).

Naturally, pharmaceutical manufacturers are keen that their products produce the minimum number of side-effects, so they develop their drugs to be as specific as possible for the intended targets. As a general principle, the more specific a drug is for an intended target then the fewer side-effects will be produced. In the case of *salbutamol*, it is designated as a β_2 adrenergic receptor agonist, which means that it will bind more specifically to β_2 adrenergic receptors than any other sub-class in the adrenergic family. However, the differences in shape between the β_1 and the β_2 adrenergic receptor are relatively small, so inevitably a drug that targets one will also inadvertently bind to and interact with the other. This unintended interaction accounts for most of the other side-effects of *salbutamol* mentioned above.

KEY FACT

The more specific a drug is for its intended target, the fewer **side-effects** it is likely to produce.

The example discussed above of how *salbutamol* can cause side-effects can be applied to many of the drugs that target receptors. Opioid pain-killers such as *morphine* and *codeine* target opioid receptors in the pain pathways of the central nervous system but also bind to receptors in the gut, which reduces its motility. Consequently, constipation is a frequent side-effect of most opioid drugs.

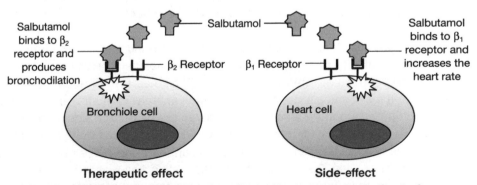

Figure 3.5 Salbutamol produces the side-effect of tachycardia by binding to β_1 receptors on the heart as well as its target β_2 receptors.

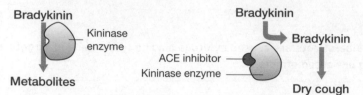

Figure 3.6 ACE inhibitors block kininases that break down bradykinin. This now accumulates and irritates the bronchioles, causing a dry cough.

Example of side-effects 2: ACE inhibitors and dry cough

Many of our most common drugs such as ACE inhibitors, NSAIDs and statins bind to the active site of key enzymes and block their action. This produces beneficial results such as lowering blood pressure, relieving inflammatory pain and reducing blood cholesterol. Unfortunately, these enzymes are often members of families of enzymes and drugs can stray off target, hit other members of the family and cause side-effects.

ACE inhibitors such as *captopril*, *enalapril* and *ramipril* are widely prescribed anti-hypertensive drugs. As we shall see in Chapter 5, these drugs bind to an enzyme called **angiotensin converting enzyme** (ACE) and inhibit its action of converting **angiotensin I** to **angiotensin II**. By interfering with various processes such as sodium balance, this reduces blood pressure. However, in the lungs there are **kininases**, enzymes similar to ACE, and these metabolise a chemical called **bradykinin** into its metabolites. Unfortunately ACE inhibitors also have an affinity for this enzyme and can inhibit its action, resulting in the build-up of bradykinin, which has an irritant action on the lining of the lungs. This is what causes the dry cough that prevents some people from using ACE inhibitors (Figure 3.6).

Example of side-effects 3: *verapamil* and constipation

As we saw in Chapter 2, ion channels are popular targets for drugs that include local anaesthetics, drugs used for mental health problems, anti-hypertensives and drugs used to treat heart **arrhythmias** (irregular heartbeats). Because ion channels are present in every cell, tissue and organ of the body, a drug that not only hits its intended target but blocks ion channels elsewhere in the body, will inevitably result in side-effects.

Verapamil is used both for hypertension and also for arrhythmias. It works by inhibiting the opening of **calcium channels** in various cells of the heart and preventing Ca^{2+} entering those cells. This has the effect of slowing the heart and maintaining a steady rhythm. Unfortunately, calcium channels are widely distributed around the body, as well as on the heart. The smooth muscle cells that surround all of the **hollow organs** of the body, such as the blood vessels and the gut, contract in response to calcium entering those cells. This means that if the calcium channels on those cells are blocked with a Ca^{2+} blocking drug such as *verapamil*, this interferes with contraction and promotes dilation. Some anti-hypertensive drugs such as *diltiazem* exploit this action by causing dilation of the

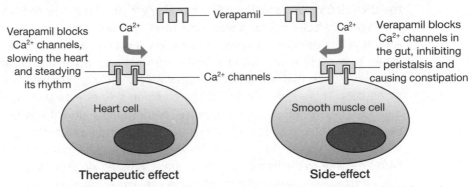

Figure 3.7 *Verapamil* blocks calcium channels in the gut, inhibiting peristalsis and causing constipation.

peripheral arterioles and reducing blood pressure – as we will see in Chapter 5. Unfortunately, blocking contraction of smooth muscle in the gut has less beneficial results because it inhibits **peristalsis** (the rhythmic muscular contraction that pushes food and partially digested material from one end of the digestive system to the other). It is little wonder, therefore, that many of our Ca^{2+} blocking drugs have constipation as one of their main side-effects (Figure 3.7).

A QUICK RECAP on side-effects caused by drugs hitting the wrong target

- Drugs bind mainly to proteins, mainly by shape, like a key fits a lock.
- Some proteins are members of families of similarly shaped proteins and drugs can bind to other members of the protein family, as well as their intended target.
- When drugs bind to an unintended target they can cause unwanted side-effects.
- Adrenaline has many sub-classes of receptor so drugs have the potential to bind to unintended adrenaline receptors and produce unwanted side-effects.
- *Salbutamol* targets β_2 adrenergic receptors in the lungs, but can also bind to β_1 receptors on the heart and cause tachycardia.
- Drugs can inadvertently block an unintended enzyme. For example, ACE inhibitors can inhibit bradykinin-degrading enzymes in the lungs, resulting in a dry cough.
- Drugs can inadvertently block an unintended ion channel. For example, *verapamil* can block calcium channels in the wall of the digestive system resulting in a reduction in peristalsis, thus causing constipation.

How drugs can cause side-effects 3: drugs that are intrinsically hazardous

Some drugs, especially those used to treat cancers, work by inflicting damage on rapidly dividing cells. They do this by a variety of means, including sticking together the DNA strands, fragmenting DNA, blocking enzymes essential to DNA synthesis, paralysing the cells' **microtubules** (fine tubes that form a sort of cellular skeleton). Although this damage is targeted at rapidly dividing cancerous cells, inevitably other cells receive unwanted attention from these quite unpleasant drugs – especially those that are dividing legitimately such as **epithelial** cells and white blood cells. This explains some of the common side-effects such as dry mouth, hair loss, gastro-intestinal disturbance, **neutropaenia** (low levels of circulating **neutrophils**), etc. In addition to interfering with normal cell division, many of the anti-cancer drugs are intrinsically toxic and need careful monitoring as they can cause damage to the heart, nervous tissue, lungs and kidneys. Nausea and vomiting are frequent side-effects of anti-cancer treatment and are very distressing to patients. Some drugs, such as *cisplatin* and *cyclophosphamide*, are notorious for this problem.

Why would anyone want to use such dangerous drugs?

Cancer is a very serious, life-threatening disease and some of the drugs used to treat it have a fairly brutal mechanism of action on the body, so it is not surprising that their side-effects are among the most unpleasant of all drug groups. However, as they can be life-saving or at least life-prolonging, their benefit generally outweighs the disagreeable side-effects they may cause.

> **Epithelial cells** are those that line the parts of the body exposed to the external environment, including the skin, lungs and digestive tract. Lining cells inside the body such as those that line blood vessels are called **endothelial** cells.

3.3   Drug interactions

Many patients, especially the elderly, may have multiple health problems that require a combination of drugs. Patients may be suffering from diabetes, rheumatic pains, hypertension, fluid retention and digestive problems and, as a consequence, different drugs may be prescribed for each of these disorders. Multiple prescribing, or **polypharmacy** as it is sometimes called, can cause some of the drugs to interact with one another and this can cause additional side-effects for the patient. Drug interaction is not a rare occurrence and a glance at Appendix 1 of the *British National Formulary* will show the extent of the problem with over 80 pages listing how one drug can interact with another.

Interactions between drugs will either increase or decrease the activity of one of those drugs. However, to be worthy of interest, an interaction must be of clinical significance. For example, drug A may marginally decrease the activity of drug B but if this does not produce any measurable change in the therapeutic effectiveness of drug B or change its side-effects profile, then its interaction is of little or no clinical relevance. Those drugs where a small change in concentration can have severe consequences are more likely to have serious interactions. These drugs include some of the **anticoagulants** (anticlotting drugs) and **anti-arrhythmics** (drugs to restore normal heart rhythm).

> **Polypharmacy** literally means 'many drugs' and is a term used when a patient has been prescribed several different drugs. This is especially a problem for the elderly who often have multiple problems, each requiring its own range of drugs.

Interactions involving hepatic P450 enzymes

Cytochrome P450 enzymes in the liver specialise in metabolising (breaking down) unwanted substances – including many drugs. When an unwanted substance, which might be a potential toxin, is present in the blood, the liver will respond by increasing the production of P450 enzymes specific to that substance. This is the basis for P450 interactions. Some drugs can induce an increase in enzyme activity that results in other substances being metabolised more quickly, and these substances can include other drugs. This means that when the activity of certain P450 enzymes is increased, those drugs that are substrates for those enzymes are metabolised more quickly and this decreases their bioavailability (Figure 3.8).

Like most other enzymes, P450 hepatic enzymes can be inhibited by drugs and other substances. When particular P450 enzymes are inhibited and their activity decreases, those drugs that are substrates for those enzymes are metabolised more slowly and this increases their bioavailability (Figure 3.9).

Examples of drugs that inhibit P450 enzymes are given in Table 3.2, together with some of the drugs whose circulating levels are increased as a consequence.

Examples of drugs that increase P450 enzyme activity are given in Table 3.3, together with some of the drugs whose circulating levels are reduced as a consequence.

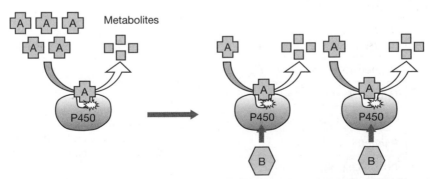

Figure 3.8 The effect of drug B inducing the production of additional P450 enzymes is to increase the overall rate of metabolism and so decrease levels of drug A.

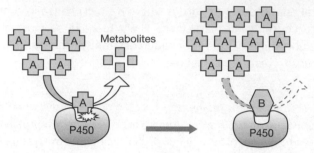

Figure 3.9 Drug A is normally broken down to its metabolites by a P450 enzyme. The effect of drug B inhibiting that enzyme is to increase levels of drug A.

Table 3.2 Examples of drugs that inhibit P450 enzymes and so increase the circulating levels of other drugs

Drugs that inhibit drug metabolising enzymes	Drugs affected by inhibition (circulating levels are increased)
Cimetidine (reduces stomach acid)	*Amiodarone* (anti-arrhythmic) *Pethidine* (pain reliever) *Warfarin* (anticoagulant)
Corticosteroids (anti-inflammatory)	*Amitriptyline* (antidepressant)
Ciprofloxacin (antibacterial)	*Theophylline* (asthma reliever)
Phenelzine (antidepressant)	*Pethidine* (pain reliever)

Table 3.3 Examples of drugs that increase P450 enzyme activity and so decrease the circulating levels of other drugs

Drugs that increase the activity of drug metabolising enzymes	Drugs affected by the increase (circulating levels are reduced)
Phenobarbital (anti-epileptic)	*Warfarin* (anticoagulant) Oral contraceptives Corticosteroids (anti-inflammatory) *Ciclosporin* (immunosuppressant)
Rifampicin (antibacterial)	
Griseofulvin (antifungal)	
Phenytoin (anti-epileptic)	
Ethanol (alcoholic drinks)	
Carbamazepine (anti-epileptic)	

> **DID YOU KNOW...** that many other substances can cause interactions besides drugs? The herbal remedy St John's wort (*Hypericum perforatum*) is a strong inducer of P450 enzymes while grapefruit juice acts as an inhibitor and increases levels of various drugs, including the cholesterol-lowering drugs *simvastatin* and *atorvastatin* plus the anti-arrhythmic, *amiodarone* (see Appendix 1 of the BNF for a full list of these interactions).

Other mechanisms of drug interactions

There are many other mechanisms whereby drugs interact, for example, the beta-blockers, a group that includes *atenolol*, *bisoprolol* and *propranolol* compete with *salbutamol* for the beta-2 receptors in the lungs. Beta-blockers work primarily by blocking β_1 adrenergic receptors on the heart from the stimulatory action of adrenaline and noradrenaline. This has the effect of reducing the workload of the heart, and easing the symptoms of angina and heart failure. Beta-blockers target the β_1 adrenergic receptors on the heart but lacking total specificity, also bind to the β_2 receptors in the lungs and block them, not only from adrenaline but also from the bronchodilator *salbutamol*. This means that for any asthmatic who suffers an asthma attack, their inhaler will be rendered ineffective because their β_2 adrenergic receptors, the targets for *salbutamol*, are all blocked by beta-blockers (Figure 3.10). This side-effect can be very serious in asthmatics; it is so serious that beta-blockers are **contra-indicated** (should not be administered) for patients with asthma.

The anticoagulant drug *warfarin* is susceptible to interactions with both antibiotics and common foods. Antibacterial drugs such as *rifampicin*, used to treat digestive infections, also reduce the population of friendly bacteria in the large intestine. Normally, these friendly bacteria produce **vitamin K** that acts as a substrate for the liver enzyme **vitamin K reductase** in the biochemical pathway that produces various circulating coagulation proteins. *Warfarin* competes with vitamin K for the active site of vitamin K reductase and so reduces the production of coagulation

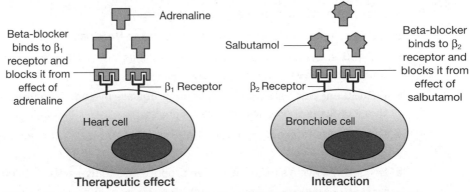

Figure 3.10 Beta-blockers can result in bronchospasm by binding to β_2 receptors on the bronchioles and blocking them from the bronchodilatory action of *salbutamol*.

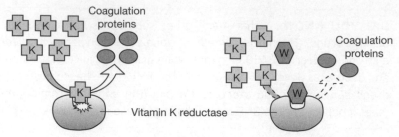

Figure 3.11 Vitamin K (K) and *warfarin* (W) compete for the active site of the enzyme vitamin K reductase. Fluctuating levels of vitamin K affect the ability of *warfarin* to compete for the active site.

proteins (Figure 3.11). As *rifampicin* causes vitamin K levels to fall, *warfarin* has a greater opportunity to bind to and block vitamin K reductase, further reducing the production of coagulation proteins and increasing the chance of haemorrhage. Logically, if a fall in vitamin K levels increases coagulation, a rise in vitamin K levels should have the opposite effect. This is why patients on *warfarin* are warned against suddenly consuming large amounts of leafy green vegetables such as cabbage, broccoli and sprouts, because it may cause inappropriate clotting.

Drugs with a similar therapeutic activity can cause problems if administered together. This is called **additive** or **summative action**, and an example would be the joint administration of the anticoagulants *warfarin* and *aspirin*. Although their mechanisms of action are different, when given together they can result in an increased risk of haemorrhage and can be especially problematical if the patient develops a **peptic ulcer**, which can cause bleeding into the stomach. Another herbal remedy worth mentioning here is the maidenhair tree, *Ginkgo biloba*, that is reputed to improve cerebral circulation. As the **ginkgolides** contained in its leaves have an anticoagulant action, it would be inadvisable to use this herb with either *aspirin* or *warfarin* because of the potential additive effect causing unwanted bleeding.

There are lots more interactions; have a look in Appendix 1 of the BNF.

A QUICK RECAP on how drugs interact

- P450 enzymes in the liver metabolise drugs.

- Some drugs can either increase or decrease P450 activity.

- If P450 enzymes are increased, some drugs are metabolised more quickly and this reduces those drugs' bioavailability.

- If P450 enzymes are inhibited, some drugs are metabolised more slowly and this increases those drugs' bioavailability.

- Other drugs interact by competing for the same receptor, e.g. *salbutamol* and *propranolol*.

- Drugs that have a similar effect can produce an additive effect if taken together.

- Herbal remedies and even common foodstuffs, such as grapefruit juice and cabbage, can interact with drugs.

3.4 Factors that determine the correct dosage of drugs

A key objective in the administration of a drug is to produce a therapeutically appropriate level of that drug in the blood and tissues. There are two key factors that affect the blood concentration: the rate of administration and the rate of elimination. Ideally, where treatment is to last several days or weeks, the rate of administration should match the rate of elimination so that the amount of drug in the body remains fairly constant.

ANOTHER WAY TO PICTURE THIS

Getting the right levels of drug in the patient is rather like running a bath with the plug missing. Water is coming in via the taps (drug administration) and water is leaving via the plughole (drug elimination). The only way to keep the level constant is to ensure that water is going in at the same rate as it is leaving the bath

Generally, for each individual drug, the rate of elimination is reasonably constant as they are continuously metabolised by the liver and excreted by the kidneys. Administration, on the other hand, tends to be periodic, either by regular injections or by ingestion. Parenteral administration resolves this problem with continuous delivery. Patient-controlled analgesia (PCA), where the patient has control of the rate of delivery of pain-relieving drugs, is designed to achieve a reasonably steady state.

Once the rate of elimination has been determined, it is possible to calculate the dose required to reach therapeutic levels. This level of drug in the body is important because if levels are too low, the drug will be ineffective and if levels are too high, the drug may be toxic. There are two terms used to describe these levels . . .

1 **Minimum effective concentration** (MEC). This is the minimum amount of drug that will produce the desired therapeutic effect

2 **Maximum safe concentration** (MSC). This is the maximum amount of drug that can be tolerated before it starts to produce toxic effects

The general principle of correct drug administration is to ensure that the level of circulating drug is maintained between these two values for the period determined to be required for the course of treatment. Figure 3.12 shows a correctly administered enteral drug whose average concentration in the blood always remains between the MEC and the MSC. After each dose, levels rise and fall as the drug is metabolised and eliminated by the body. However, before the level of drug falls below the MEC, another dose is administered to top up the level.

The difference between the MEC and MSC is sometimes called the **therapeutic window** and the calculated ratio of MEC to MSC defines the **therapeutic index** (TI) by the following formula:

$$\text{Therapeutic index (TI)} = \frac{\text{MSC}}{\text{MEC}}$$

65

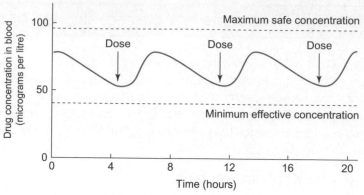

Figure 3.12 A correctly administered drug maintains levels between the minimum effective concentration and the maximum safe concentration.

This means that the larger the therapeutic index, the less likelihood there is of adverse reactions if the normal dose is exceeded for any reason. However, it cannot be stressed strongly enough that there is no room for any error in the administration of drugs – even when a drug has a wide therapeutic index. Drugs that have a very narrow therapeutic index, such as *digoxin*, *theophylline* and *warfarin*, need very careful monitoring indeed to ensure that levels are kept tightly controlled within the therapeutic index.

Establishing the therapeutic index does not tell us how much drug to administer because it takes no account of the rate of elimination. The rate at which a drug is eliminated is quantified by its **half-life** ($T^1/_2$), the time it takes for the concentration of a drug to decrease by half, from (say) 100 micrograms per litre to 50 micrograms per litre. The longer the half-life, the longer the drug will remain in the circulation, and vice versa. The shorter the half-life, the more frequently a drug needs to be administered, and vice versa. Look at the two drugs in Figure 3.13.

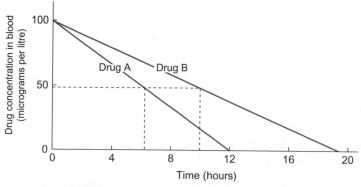

Figure 3.13 Differences in the rate of metabolism or elimination give drugs A and B different half-lives.

It can be seen from Figure 3.13 that the time taken for drug A and drug B to fall from a plasma concentration of 100 micrograms per litre to 50 micrograms per litre (i.e. by half) is different. $T^1/_2$ for drug A is around 6 hours while $T^1/_2$ for drug B is around 10 hours. If 100 micrograms per litre is the desired plasma concentration for the drug, then drug A will need to be delivered more frequently. However, if it has a larger therapeutic index, a larger dose of drug A may be safely given at less frequent intervals. Fortunately for those who administer drugs, these calculations are done in the development process by the drug manufacturers and it is then the responsibility of clinical staff to ensure that they administer the correct dosage of the drug in accordance with current recommendations.

A QUICK RECAP on factors that determine the correct dosage of drugs

- For drugs that are to be prescribed over a period of days or weeks, the delivery of the drug needs to match the rate of metabolism and elimination.

- The level of drugs in the body needs to be kept above the minimum effective concentration (MEC) and below the maximum safe concentration (MSC).

- The difference between the MEC and the MSC is called the therapeutic window and its calculated ratio is the therapeutic index (TI).

- The half-life of a drug ($T^1/_2$) is the time it takes for the concentration of a drug to fall by one half.

RUNNING WORDS

Here are some of the technical terms that were included in this chapter. Read them one by one and tick them off when you are sure that you understand them.

Additive action p. 64
Angiotensin-converting enzyme p. 58
Angiotensin I p. 58
Angiotensin II p. 58
Anti-arrhythmics p. 61
Anticoagulants p. 61
Arrhythmias p. 58
Bile p. 51
Bioavailability p. 50
Bradykinin p. 58
Bronchodilation p. 54
Buffer p. 50
Calcium channels p. 58
Chronic p. 45
Coagulation p. 54
Contra-indicated p. 63
Corticosteroids p. 48
Cytochrome P450 p. 50
Dose-related p. 54
Endothelial p. 60
Enteral p. 47
Epithelial p. 60
Erythropoietin p. 51
First-pass metabolism p. 50

Ginkgolides p. 64
Haemorrhage p. 54
Half-life p. 66
Hepatic portal vein p. 49
Hepatic vein p. 50
Hollow organs p. 58
Hypotension p. 53
Intramuscular p. 47
Intravenously p. 47
Jejunum p. 47
Kininases p. 58
Maximum safe concentration p. 65
Mesenteric artery p. 49
Metabolism p. 46
Metabolites p. 51
Microsomal enzyme p. 50
Microtubules p. 60
Minimum effective concentration p. 65
Neutropaenia p. 60
Neutrophils p. 60
Oestrogen p. 48
Palpitations p. 56
Parenteral p. 47

Patient-controlled analgesia p. 48
Peptic ulcer p. 64
Peristalsis p. 59
Polypharmacy p. 60
Pro-drugs p. 51
Side-effects p. 52
Smooth muscle cells p. 55
Sub-lingual p. 48
Subcutaneous p. 48
Summative action p. 64
Suppositories p. 48
Sympathomimetic p. 56
Tachycardia p. 54
Therapeutic index p. 65
Therapeutic window p. 65
Topical p. 47
Transdermal p. 48
Tremor p. 56
Vasoconstriction p. 55
Vasodilation p. 55
Vitamin K p. 63
Vitamin K reductase p. 63

REFERENCES AND FURTHER RECOMMENDED READING

Coleman M. (2006) *Drug Metabolism*. Wiley-Blackwell.

Your turn to try

Now you have finished reading the chapter it's time to find out how much you have learned. Side-effects, drug metabolism and interactions are important aspects of pharmacology so it is important that you understand these topics.

The answers to these questions are at the end of the book on page 283.

1 Name a drug or group of drugs that can cause unwanted effects by tipping the balance too far as they try to restore homoeostasis.

2 If we say the effect of a drug is **dose related**, what do we mean?

3 What is the effect of adrenaline binding to a β_1 receptor on the heart?

4 Why may salbutamol, a β_2 receptor agonist, cause tachycardia?

5 ACE inhibitors such as *captopril* can accidently bind to and block kininase enzymes in the bronchioles – how might this cause the side-effect of dry cough?

6 How may calcium channel blockers such as *verapamil* cause constipation?

7 Why may anticancer drugs affect circulating levels of white blood cells?

8 Name the three major routes of drug administration.

9 Describe the passage of drugs from the digestive system to the circulation.

10 Why can insulin not be administered orally?

11 Why can *glyceryl trinitrate* (GTN) not be administered orally?

12 What is first-pass metabolism?

13 If P450 enzymes are inhibited by a drug is it more likely that other drugs will increase or decrease in their bioavailability?

14 What is the therapeutic window?

15 What is the half-life of a drug?

Answers to questions on page 45

1 Proteins.
2 ATP is the energy molecule that powers biochemical reactions in cells.
3 Lipids.
4 Hormones, neurotransmitters and mediators.
5 Antagonists.

Part 2

The major drug groups

Chapter 4

The cardiovascular system (1)

Drugs used in the management of coronary artery disease

AIMS

By the time you have finished the chapter you will understand:

1 The **physiology** – the basic anatomy and physiology of the circulatory system.
2 The **pathology** – coronary artery disease and its consequences.
3 The **pharmacology** – action of the major drug groups used to prevent and to treat coronary artery disease.

CONTENTS

The chapter contains some brief case studies and finishes off with some self-test questions, so you can make sure that you have understood the physiology, pathology and pharmacology of this important area.

> ### IN PRACTICE
>
> You will find that coronary artery disease is depressingly common, especially among the elderly and particularly those from poorer, underprivileged back-grounds. The disease itself can take many forms from mild angina through to congestive heart failure and it is often associated with other chronic dis-eases such as diabetes and hypertension. In any branch of adult medicine you will undoubtedly encounter patients with heart problems, so you need to understand the nature of the disease and also the many different types of drugs used in its treatment.

Introduction

Let's start off with a not very cheerful statistic: according to the UK Statistics Authority, Coronary Artery Disease (CAD) is the cause of more deaths in the UK than any other disease. This is a sad (but true) fact - and it's almost certain that most of us will know of a relative or acquaintance who has had a heart attack. Fortunately, the chances of surviving a heart attack have been greatly improved in recent years and many people are alive today thanks to the excellent standard of treatment by paramedics and emergency care teams, not to mention advances in drug therapy. You can see, therefore, how important it is for all clinical practi-tioners to have a basic knowledge of the circulatory system, the nature of coronary artery disease and also familiarity with the common drugs used in its prevention and treatment.

This chapter follows a format that will become familiar to you as you read the following chapters in Part 2. Firstly, we make sure that you understand the basic anatomy and physiology of the circulatory system. Secondly, we help you to under-stand something about the pathology of coronary artery disease, its causes and its consequences. Finally, we put this knowledge to good use when we explore how the main groups of anticoagulant, anti-anginal and lipid-lowering drugs work to help to prevent and treat this disease. We also include a brief section of some common but fairly specialised drugs used to treat abnormal heart rhythms.

In this and the next chapter you will find that several drugs have more than one indication, in other words they are used for more than one type of cardiovascular disease. For example, some of the beta-blockers such as *propranolol*, *atenolol*, *bisoprolol*, etc., are used to alleviate angina, lower high blood pressure, help with heart failure and prevent arrhythmias (abnormal heart beat) - not to mention relieving various symptoms associated with anxiety. To save repetition, we will just explain the action of each drug once rather than repeat its action for each pathology.

> **Arrhythmias** such as palpitations can be annoying but not life threatening whereas others, especially after a heart attack, can be very serious indeed. The term *arrhythmia* can refer to an irregular heart beat or one that is abnormally slow or fast.

WHERE ARE WE STARTING FROM?

In the next two chapters we shall look at the circulatory system and its associated pathologies in some detail – as well as the drugs that are used to treat those pathologies. *Introducing Pharmacology* is primarily (as the title implies) a book about pharmacology so we cannot explain all of the anatomy, physiology and pathologies of the circulatory system. We will, however, cover enough of the basics of these topics in Chapters 4 and 5 to enable you to understand the action of the main drugs used to treat cardiovascular disease. The general physiology and pathophysiology books in your College or University library will help you to explore the subject in more depth. Some suggestions for recommended reading are provided at the end of this chapter.

Do we really need two chapters just devoted to the circulatory system? Yes indeed you do. An understanding of the circulatory system is essential to anyone training or working in clinical practice. Think how often nurses and doctors take a patient's blood pressure or pulse. Also, if you do not understand the basic physiology of the circulatory system you will never understand the action of the drugs used to treat cardiovascular diseases.

Let's start off with a short quiz to find out how much you know before we begin:

1 Point to your heart – is it on the left or right side of your chest?

2 Do arteries carry blood to or from the heart?

3 How many chambers are there in the heart?

4 Starting from the heart, arrange these blood vessels in the order that the blood flows – capillaries, arteries and veins.

5 What is the name of the arteries that supply the heart muscle with blood?

Answers are at the end of the chapter on page 108.

How did you do? If you struggled, make sure that you read Section 4.1 carefully to ensure that you understand the basic physiology of the circulatory system.

4.1   The physiology of the cardiovascular system

The circulatory system is made up of the heart, the blood vessels and blood and can be thought of as the body's internal transport system, carrying messages and materials from one part of the body to another. The circulatory system is also central to maintaining the stability of the internal environment, those processes that control nutrient levels and waste disposal as well as water and temperature regulation. The need for an internal transport system arose hundreds of millions of years ago when single-celled organisms started to aggregate into larger, multi-cellular organisms. Their increase in size then became limited by the rate at which nutrients and gasses could be obtained from the environment by simple diffusion. The development of a simple circulation meant that nutrients and gasses could be collected by specialist organs such as the gut and gills* and then transported to all of the cells of the body. We might speculate that without the development of the circulatory system, animal life as we know it today would not exist – including perhaps ourselves!

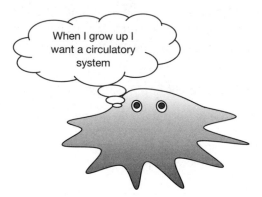

Overview of the circulatory system

The circulatory system is the main transport system of the body, transporting nutrients, respiratory gasses, wastes, hormones, immune cells and clotting proteins around the body in the blood. It also has other functions, such as temperature control and acidity regulation that are essential for the well-being of the individual. In the context of pharmacology, it is also the system that transports most of our

---

* The move from single-celled to multicellular animals probably happened in the sea, so these primitive animals would have had gills rather than lungs to collect oxygen.

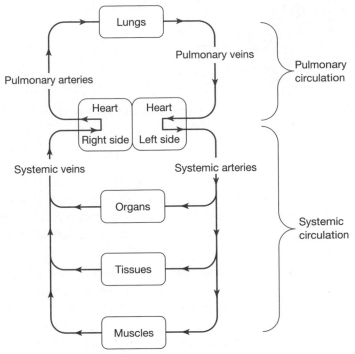

Figure 4.1 Schematic diagram of the circulatory system showing the pulmonary and systemic systems.

drugs around the body, from the site of administration to the tissues targeted by those drugs.

The circulatory system is divided into two parts, the **pulmonary system** supplying the lungs and the **systemic system** supplying the rest of the body (Figure 4.1). At the centre of both systems is the heart, a large, muscular pump which beats 70 or so times each minute from a few weeks after conception to the last minute of the individual's life. A simple calculation indicates that by the age of 70, the heart has beat over 2.5 billion times. Although it is a single organ, the heart is not a single pump but two separate pumps joined together and beating in unison. The right-hand pump sends blood to the pulmonary circulation, around the lungs from where it returns to the left-hand heart pump. From the left-hand pump the blood is sent around the systemic circulation to the tissues and organs of the body. The blood then returns to the right-hand pump from where it is again sent around the pulmonary circulation.

Blood vessels

Blood vessels are the body's plumbing system, carrying blood from one part of the circulatory system to another. These vessels can be divided broadly into three types: **arteries, veins,** and **capillaries**, each having a different structure and function.

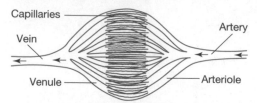

Figure 4.2 Relationship between the blood vessels of the arterial and venous system. The arrows indicate the direction of blood flow.

- **Arteries.** These thick-walled, muscular tubes carry high-pressure blood away from the heart, supplying blood to organs and muscles where they branch into smaller arteries called **arterioles**. The body can adjust the diameter of the arterioles to control blood pressure – as discussed in more detail in Chapter 5.

- **Veins.** These have thinner walls than arteries and carry low-pressure blood back to the heart. Small one-way valves help to keep the blood moving in one direction. Veins are larger in diameter than their arterial counterparts and over 60 per cent of the body's blood is retained in the veins at any one time. The tiniest of veins, where they emerge from tissues and organs, are called **venules**.

- **Capillaries.** These are the smallest of the blood vessels, being only one cell thick and they permeate nearly every cubic millimetre of every tissue of the body. The walls of arteries and veins are too thick to allow gasses and nutrients to cross their walls, so it is in the capillaries where the exchange of materials between the blood and the body's cells takes place.

Figure 4.2 shows the relationship of the various blood vessels to the circulatory system.

CASE STUDY

Harry is admitted to A & E complaining of severe chest pains and difficulty breathing but an ECG confirms that he has not suffered a heart attack. Further tests indicate a pulmonary thromboembolism – a blood clot in the lungs. The consultant diagnoses that the problem originated with a deep vein thrombosis (DVT) in Harry's leg. Explain how a DVT in the leg might cause problems in the lungs.

Comment on case study A blood clot that forms in the veins of the leg (deep vein thrombosis) can often cause a pulmonary thromboembolism – a blood clot in the lungs. The blood clot travels in the ever-widening veins to the right side of the heart where it enters the pulmonary circulation and soon blocks one of the ever-narrowing pulmonary arteries, causing chest pain and difficulty in breathing.

The circulatory system and gas exchange

As we saw in Chapter 1, glucose and fatty acids are broken down in the body's cells to produce adenosine triphosphate (ATP) and this requires a good supply of oxygen. Carbon dioxide is a waste produced during cellular energy production and needs to be removed from the cells, otherwise its accumulation could inhibit metabolic activity. The transport of oxygen to the tissues and the removal of carbon dioxide is a very important function of the circulatory system and must be maintained constantly throughout the life of the individual. Any disease or trauma that interferes with the transport of gasses, especially oxygen, quickly results in problems, the death of cells and even the demise of the individual.

If you refer to Figure 4.2 (above) you will see that blood constantly flows between the pulmonary and systemic circulation. In the pulmonary circulation, the blood collects oxygen, then travels via the systemic circulation to the muscles, organs and tissues where the oxygen is released to the cells in order that they may produce energy. During the process of energy production, carbon dioxide, which is produced in the cells, is collected by the blood and transported to the pulmonary system where it is disposed of into the atmosphere via the lungs.

The heart

Ask most people where their heart is situated and they will point vaguely to the left side of their chest. The heart is in fact situated in the centre of the chest, directly under the **sternum** (breastbone) but on a slightly tilted axis so that the lower pointed part or **apex** is on the left-hand side. This means that when the heart is beating strongly, the heart beat can be heard more clearly on the left-hand side where you can also feel it by placing your fingers just to the left of the sternum.

The structure of the heart

The heart consists of four chambers, two **atria** and two **ventricles**. Blood arriving at the heart from the **vena-cava** and the **pulmonary veins** first enters the atria from where it passes into the ventricles, which are the main pumping chambers of the heart. When the left and right ventricles contract, blood is forced into the **aorta** and **pulmonary arteries** respectively. Separating the atria and the ventricles are one-way valves, collectively known as the **atrioventricular valves**. Another set of valves called the **semilunar valves** separate the ventricles from the arteries. Figure 4.3 shows the general structure of the heart and Figure 4.4 shows the route by which the blood flows through it. Most of the force that pumps the blood out of the heart comes from contraction of the thick muscular wall of the heart – the **myocardium**. The myocardium consists almost entirely of cardiac muscle cells which are unique to the heart, being found in no other part of the body. As might be expected in a muscle mass that may beat continuously for over 70 years, energy supply is of prime importance and the cardiac muscle cells are rich in ATP-producing mitochondria.

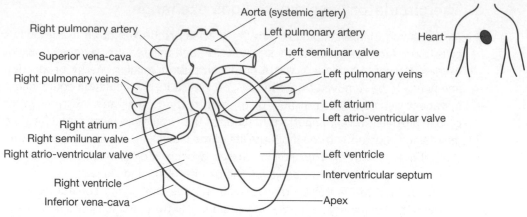

Figure 4.3 Front view of the heart in section. The small diagram to the right shows the position of the heart in the thoracic cavity.

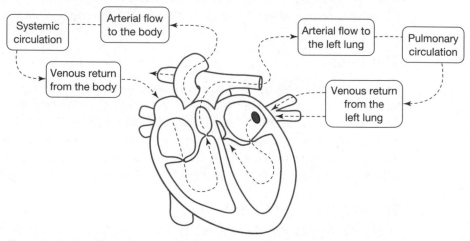

Figure 4.4 Simplified diagram of blood flow through the heart, the systemic circulation and the pulmonary circulation. Left pulmonary blood flow only is shown for clarity.

The pumping cycle of the heart can be divided into two stages, **diastole** (pronounced *die-ass-toe-lee*) when the heart is relaxed and filling with blood and **systole** (pronounced *sis-toe-lee*) when the heart is contracting and pumping blood into the arteries. We will learn more about systole and diastole in Chapter 5 when we examine the control of the heart and how the body regulates blood pressure.

Myocardium is the middle layer of the heart wall and comprises cardiac muscle cells. As the cells contract, a wave of contraction in the myocardium pumps blood out of the heart into the arteries.

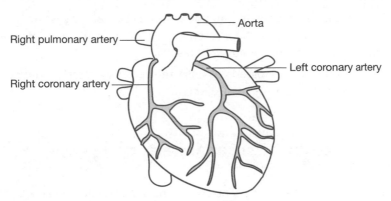

Figure 4.5 The coronary circulation. Blood vessels emerging from the aorta supply the heart muscle with blood, nutrients and oxygen.

The blood supply to the myocardium

Most people would assume that the heart obtained its oxygen and nutrients from the blood that is constantly being pumped through the atria and ventricles. However, if you look back at Figure 4.5 you will see that the myocardium, the muscular wall of the heart, is quite thick, too thick in fact to obtain its nutrients and oxygen by simple diffusion. To resolve this problem, the heart has its own blood supply via its own blood vessels and this is called the **coronary circulation** (Figure 4.5). The blood supply for the coronary circulation comes from the two coronary arteries which emerge from the base of the aorta. These coronary arteries wrap themselves around the heart, the right coronary artery supplying the right atrium and right ventricle and the left coronary artery supplying the left atrium and left ventricle. The arteries are initially visible on the surface of the heart but then dive into the heart muscle and divide into arterioles and capillaries.

DID YOU KNOW . . . why the arteries of the heart are called coronary arteries? It is because they are vaguely shaped like a crown worn by the Queen. This is where the word *coronation* comes from. Turn Figure 4.6 upside down and you will see. However, if you think the inverted arteries look more like reindeer antlers than a crown - you are not alone!

A QUICK RECAP on the circulatory system

- The main function of the circulatory system is the transport of materials around the body. Of special importance is the transport of oxygen from the lungs to the cells of the tissues.

- There are two parts of the circulatory system - the pulmonary circulation and the systemic circulation.

- There are three main types of blood vessels - arteries, veins and capillaries. All of these vessels transport blood but it is in the capillaries that exchange takes place between the blood and the cells.

- The heart is the double driving pump of the circulatory system – the left half pumps blood through the systemic circulation and the right half pumps blood through the pulmonary circulation.
- The heart has its own blood vessels – the coronary arteries that supply blood to the heart muscle – myocardium.

4.2   The pathology of coronary artery disease

Atherosclerosis in the coronary arteries is the principle cause of angina, **myocardial infarction** (heart attack) and heart failure. In the **carotid** arteries that supply the brain, atherosclerosis can result in stroke.

Cardiovascular disease is undoubtedly the principle cause of death in the UK and the cost of treating this problem places an enormous drain on the resources of the Health Service. Hundreds of thousands of people are afflicted with this disease; many are unable to enjoy normal activities as their lives are blighted by a pathology that is largely avoidable.

Early in the life of some individuals, the first recognisable event in the development of atherosclerosis is the formation of **fatty streaks** in the walls of the arteries. White blood cells called **macrophages** containing fat droplets of cholesterol migrate from the blood to the area just under the inner lining of the arteries called the **subendothelium**. Generally, in the healthy individual these fatty streaks remain inconspicuous but in some people they develop into **atheromata** (singular, **atheroma**) – Figures 4.6a to 4.6d.

Smooth muscle cells in the area are prompted to multiply in a disorganised and haphazard fashion and the fatty streaks enlarge into cholesterol-rich structures called atherosclerotic **plaques** that can become inflamed and unstable. In this state, the plaques can partially block the coronary arteries resulting in angina. Even worse, the plaque can rupture and a **thrombus** (blood clot) can form, blocking the coronary artery and causing a **myocardial infarction**, commonly known as a heart attack.

> **Macrophage** literally translated means 'big eater'. They are important members of the white blood cell family of immune cells with many functions, including the destruction of bacteria.

Apart from a few individuals who inherit a genetic defect in lipid regulation, most atherosclerosis is due to the lifestyle adopted by the individual. The key risk factors for cardiovascular disease are smoking, lack of exercise, eating too much saturated fat and not eating enough fruit and vegetables. Add to these risk factors, obesity and diabetes and you can almost guarantee that an individual will have heart problems. How these factors increase the risk of cardiovascular

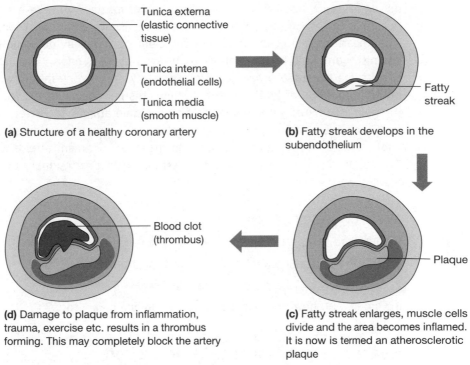

(a) Structure of a healthy coronary artery

(b) Fatty streak develops in the subendothelium

(c) Fatty streak enlarges, muscle cells divide and the area becomes inflamed. It is now is termed an atherosclerotic plaque

(d) Damage to plaque from inflammation, trauma, exercise etc. results in a thrombus forming. This may completely block the artery

Figures 4.6a to 4.6d show the development of an atherosclerotic plaque and the formation of a thrombus.

disease is quite complex but the epidemiological evidence for this is well documented.

CASE STUDY

Jim is 58, works as a truck driver and is complaining about feeling out of breath when he climbs the stairs. He is overweight, smokes and eats most of his meals in transport cafes. Given what you know about the causes of cardiovascular disease, what would you advise for Jim?

Comment on case study Jim is at risk of developing cardiovascular disease. If he is feeling out of breath, he needs to discuss this with his GP. The best advice to improve his health would be to give up smoking and change his diet by restricting his intake of saturated fats and eating plenty of fresh fruit and vegetables. He should also ensure that he takes regular exercise.

Angina pectoris

The gradual blockage of the coronary arteries by atherosclerotic plaques can result in insufficient blood and oxygen being delivered to the myocardium during exercise. Remember, whatever group of muscles you are exercising, the heart has to respond by beating faster to increase its output of blood. However, when heart muscle cells cannot get sufficient oxygen they do some clever bio-chemistry and switch on metabolic pathways that keep energy production going despite the shortage of oxygen. Unfortunately, this switch in pathways results in the production of **lactic acid** that stimulates pain neurons and this produces the pain associated with angina. In chronic **stable angina**, the arteries **occluded** (obstructed) by plaques produce a predictable, exercise-associated pain. **Unstable angina** is defined as new-onset angina, angina at rest or angina after a heart attack. The cause of unstable angina needs investigating as it may signal a thrombosis in the coronary arteries.

REALITY CHECK

Having read this part of the chapter can you now:

1 Explain the development of cardiovascular disease?

2 List the risk factors for cardiovascular disease?

3 Understand how exercise produces pain in angina pectoris?

Heart attack or myocardial infarction

When a plaque ruptures it can result in a blood clot forming around the site of rupture and this can partially or completely block the coronary artery. The heart muscle supplied by the artery is deprived of sufficient blood and oxygen and is said to be **ischaemic**. If the blood supply is not restored quickly, the myocardial muscle cells die, forming an **infarct** (area of dead tissue). This is a heart attack or myocardial infarction (MI). Damaged heart muscle can severely incapacitate the heart's ability to pump blood and eventually this may lead to **heart failure** and possibly death. The extent of the damage to the heart depends on the size and location of the artery that has been occluded. A large clot can block a large artery, which cuts off blood to a significant section of the heart muscle causing a major heart attack. A clot forming in a small terminal artery may affect only a relatively small area of muscle and the damage is potentially less serious (Figure 4.7).

IN PRACTICE

This pain experienced in a heart attack is often felt in the arm and neck as well as the chest because the pain neurons that originate in these areas all feed into the spinal cord at the same point. The brain is unable to identify the precise source of the problem so that pain is perceived as emanating from a different area to the source. This is called **referred pain**.

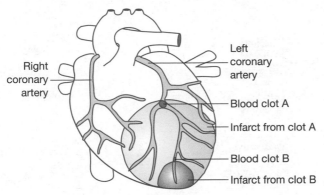

Figure 4.7 Two blood clots form in the coronary arteries. Blood clot A is large and blocks two branches of the descending left coronary artery, depriving a large area of heart muscle of blood and oxygen and severely affecting the heart's ability to pump blood. Blood clot B is smaller, blocks a minor artery and affects a smaller area of tissue.

Heart failure

The consequences of a heart attack can vary depending on the location of the thrombus, the area of heart tissue affected and most importantly, the time it takes for the paramedics to arrive. If the patient's life is saved but a significant area of the myocardium is irreparably damaged, this can eventually lead to heart failure. This is a complex process where the heart becomes more and more weakened as it attempts to maintain blood pressure and eventually becomes irreparably damaged, leading to complete failure and death.

Surgical interventions in coronary artery disease

When the problem is severe enough, surgical interventions such as **coronary artery bypass grafts** (CABG) and **percutaneous coronary interventions** (PCI) may be considered. These procedures increase the blood and therefore oxygen flow to the myocardium and so relieve angina pain and improve the heart's ability to respond to the demands of exercise. CABG involves a major operation that exposes the heart while a healthy vein or artery is removed from elsewhere in the patient and transplanted so that it bypasses the damaged coronary artery. PCI is performed using **radiographic imaging** (x-rays), to insert a long, thin wire called a **catheter** into the arterial system and directing it into the blocked coronary artery. Here, a small balloon on the end of the catheter is expanded to open up the blocked artery (Figure 4.8). A small metal cage called a **stent** is often attached to the end of the catheter and as the balloon expands so does the stent, holding open the artery and allowing blood to flow again.

While CABG and PCI can undoubtedly prolong and improve the quality of life for those with coronary artery disease, most of these patients will continue to be maintained on a regime of anticlotting drugs that we will discuss later in the chapter.

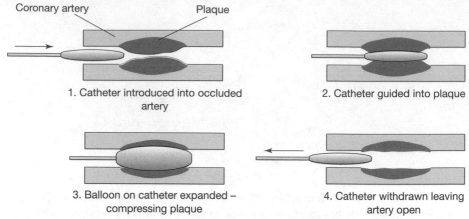

Coronary artery   Plaque

1. Catheter introduced into occluded
artery

2. Catheter guided into plaque

3. Balloon on catheter expanded –
compressing plaque

4. Catheter withdrawn leaving
artery open

Figure 4.8 Percutaneous Coronary Intervention (PCI). A balloon catheter is introduced into coronary arteries occluded by an atherosclerotic plaque. The balloon is inflated, compressing the plaque. On deflation and withdrawal, the artery is left open for blood to flow to the heart muscle.

IN PRACTICE

Could you explain to a patient or relative the difference between a coronary artery bypass graft and a percutaneous coronary intervention?

REALITY CHECK

Having read this part of the chapter can you now . . .

1 Understand the nature of coronary artery disease?

2 Explain how plaques in the coronary arteries can cause angina?

3 Explain how the rupture of a plaque can cause a heart attack?

A QUICK RECAP on coronary artery disease

● Atheromata are fatty growths that form in the wall of the coronary arteries.

● They can partially block the coronary arteries resulting in stable angina – heart pain brought on by exercise.

● Atheromata can rupture causing a thrombus (blood clot) to form in the arteries.

● The thrombus can block a coronary artery, cutting off the oxygen supply to areas of heart muscle – ischaemia.

● The continued lack of blood and oxygen can cause an infarct – death of heart muscle; this is a myocardial infarction (MI) or heart attack.

4.3   Drugs used in the treatment of coronary artery disease

Anti-angina drugs

What are we trying to do with these drugs?

The principle purpose of anti-angina drugs is to relieve the pain associated with the disease rather than treating the disease itself. This is not to say we can't help the sufferer from stable angina but the drugs used to relieve the pain do little if anything to resolve the cause of the problem, which is primarily the formation of atherosclerotic plaques in the coronary arteries.

The full treatment regime for anyone suffering from stable angina will include lifestyle changes such as giving up smoking, taking controlled exercise and eating a healthy diet that includes more fruit and vegetables and less saturated fat. To reduce the rate at which atherosclerosis develops, statins such as *atorvastatin* may be prescribed to lower cholesterol levels in the blood. Angina sufferers also run the risk of clots forming in the coronary arteries, so *aspirin* may be prescribed on a long-term basis to prevent this. The action of statins and *aspirin* will be discussed later in the chapter.

A variety of drugs are available to reduce angina pain and these include nitrates, beta-blockers and calcium channel blockers. The general aim of these drugs is to reduce the workload of the heart or dilate the coronary arteries, so delivering more oxygenated blood to the heart muscle. In this section of the chapter we will concentrate on the action of nitrates and beta-blockers and leave any detailed discussion of the calcium channel blockers until Chapter 5, when we examine their role as antihypertensive drugs.

> **KEY FACT**
>
> Anti-angina drugs relieve angina pain by reducing the workload of the heart or by increasing the blood supply to the heart muscle.

Anti-angina drugs group 1: glyceryl trinitrate and related drugs

Glyceryl trinitrate (GTN) is regularly prescribed as first-line treatment in stable angina. It is available as tablets or as a spray, both of which are used under the tongue from where the drug speedily enters the bloodstream and quickly relieves angina pain.

The action of nitrates on cells is complex but their main effect is to cause relaxation of the smooth muscle cells surrounding blood vessels and so produce vasodilation. Nitrates have various effects on different blood vessels (Figure 4.9).

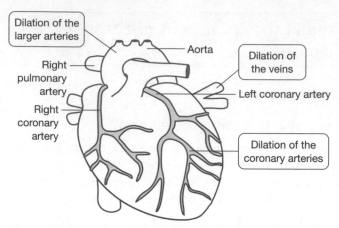

Figure 4.9 Summary of the effects of nitrates on the heart.

- **Venodilation** (dilation of the veins) reduces pressure in the veins which in turn reduces the amount of blood returning to the heart. Less blood in the ventricles when they are contracting reduces the workload of the heart.
- **Vasodilation of coronary arteries** increases blood flow to the heart muscle, bringing with it more oxygen. This reduces lactic acid production and thus pain.
- **Vasodilation of larger arteries** lowers blood pressure and reduces the amount of effort needed by the heart to pump blood out of the ventricles.

IN PRACTICE

GTN tablets are dissolved under the tongue rather than being swallowed because GTN is almost completely metabolised by the liver on its way from the digestive system to the general circulation. Dissolved under the tongue, GTN passes straight into the bloodstream. Other formulations are available that can survive passage through the liver.

GTN itself has a very short life in the circulation of around five minutes, so other formulations have been developed to provide longer-term relief from angina such as *isorbide dinitrate* and *isorbide mononitrate*. Nitrate tolerance can be a problem with these drugs as their effectiveness diminishes with long-term use.

Side-effects A drug group that causes general vasodilation can cause hypotension (low blood pressure) in some patients. Throbbing headache is another common side-effect of nitrates.

CASE STUDY

John has been suffering from angina for nearly one year. He has been using a GTN sublingual spray which seems to ease the pain that he experiences when he climbs the stairs. Recently his chest pain has returned despite the GTN. What may be the cause?

Comment on case study There are several possible causes but it could be that he is becoming tolerant to GTN and his medication needs reviewing. Another explanation could be that John's coronary arteries are becoming more occluded by the atheromata so further tests are required.

DID YOU KNOW ... that glyceryl trinitrate is the same substance as nitroglycerin, the explosive component of dynamite, invented by Alfred Nobel in the nineteenth century? Modern formulations of GTN do not carry the risk of explosion but one wonders if early pharmacists had a few close shaves with this potentially dangerous substance? GTN is also one of the oldest drugs still in use – its first appearance in the pharmacopoeia was in the 1880s.

Anti-angina drugs group 2: beta-blockers

This group of drugs is more correctly called beta-adrenoceptor antagonists in that they antagonistically block adrenergic (adrenaline) receptors. They have been in the pharmacopoeia for over 30 years and earned their inventor, Sir James Black, the Nobel Prize for Medicine in 1989 for the synthesis of *propranolol*.

Examples of this group used in the treatment of angina include *acebutolol, atenolol, bisoprolol, carvedilol, labetalol, metoprolol, nadolol, oxprenolol, pindolol, propranolol* and *timolol*. Selected members of this group of drugs are also used for hypertension and arrhythmias and heart failure.

The sympathetic neurons release the neurotransmitter noradrenaline and this stimulates β_1 adrenoceptors on the heart pacemaker cells and the heart muscle. This increases both the heart rate and contractility which in turn increases the workload of the heart and so the probability of angina-induced pain. Beta-blockers bind to and block β_1 receptors on the heart, and this reduces its responsiveness to sympathetic activity (Figure 4.10). This lowers the heart's workload to a level where the oxygen demand of the heart muscle can be met, even by the narrowed coronary arteries.

Beta-blockers also reduce blood pressure by a mechanism that is not fully understood (see Chapter 5). When BP is reduced in the aorta, this means that the heart has to beat less forcefully to push blood into the arterial system. This also helps to reduce the heart's workload and so prevents angina pain.

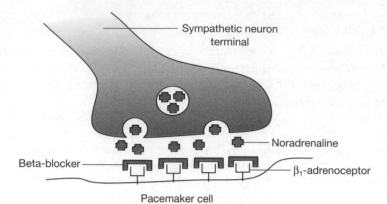

Figure 4.10 At the synapse between a sympathetic neuron and a pacemaker cell, noradrenaline is prevented from binding to its receptors by beta-blockers which lowers the heart rate.

IN PRACTICE

Beta-blockers should not be prescribed to anyone suffering from asthma. This is because these drugs can block β_2 adrenaline receptors in the bronchioles of the lungs and these receptors are the targets for bronchodilators such as *salbutamol*. If they are blocked by beta-blockers, then *salbutamol* cannot bind and activate its receptors, which could be potentially very serious for anyone having an asthma attack.

Anti-angina drugs group 3: calcium channel blockers

Examples of calcium channel blockers (CCBs) include *amlodipine, diltiazem, felodipine, nicardipine, nifedipine, nisoldipine* and *verapamil*. CCBs are a diverse group of drugs and exert their effects by different mechanisms. CCBs are a popular group of drugs that are also used in the treatment of hypertension. We will meet them again in Chapter 5 when we discuss antihypertensive drugs, and we will examine in more detail how they reduce blood pressure.

Calcium channel blockers act on calcium ion channels in the muscle cells of the heart, the conduction system of the heart and the smooth muscle cells of blood vessels. These diverse targets all result in a reduction in the pain associated with angina but by a variety of mechanisms:

1 **Reduction in heart rate.** Slowing the heart rate reduces the workload of the heart and helps to ease angina pain.

2 **Reduction in the force of contraction.** This again reduces the workload of the heart and helps to ease angina pain.

3 **Reduction in blood pressure.** Vasodilation dilates the blood vessels and this reduces blood pressure. The heart has to pump less forcefully to push blood into the arteries.

Unwanted effects These are many, including constipation (check the current BNF for a full list). Constipation is most likely caused by CCBs inhibiting contraction of the smooth muscle that encircles the gut. This reduces motility, leading to the sluggish passage of food through the gastro-intestinal system.

Anti-angina drugs group 4: potassium channel openers - *nicorandil*

Nicorandil acts on smooth muscle cells of blood vessels where it opens K^+ channels in the cell membrane, making the muscle cells more resistant to contraction. *Nicorandil* also dilates the coronary arteries thus increasing blood and oxygen supply to the myocardium. In addition to its action as a K^+ channel opener, *nicorandil* (nicotinamide nitrate) also has a nitrate-like action, acting in a similar manner to GTN.

Anti-angina drugs group 5: funny channel blockers - *ivabradine*

This is not a joke - *ivabradine* really does block a mixed Na^+/K^+ ion channel on the heart's pacemaker called the **funny channel** (who says scientists don't have a sense of humour?). This reduces the heart rate which, in turn, reduces oxygen demand by the heart muscle. This means that even with partially blocked coronary arteries, sufficient oxygenated blood can be supplied to the myocardium to prevent the muscle cells producing the lactic acid that causes angina pain.

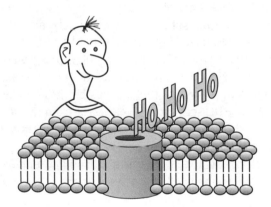

A QUICK RECAP on anti-angina drugs

- Nitrates such as *glyceryl trinitrate* reduce angina pain by general vasodilation. This reduces pressure in the arteries and ventricles and so reduces the workload of the heart. The coronary arteries are also dilated, supplying more blood and oxygen to the heart muscle.

- Beta-blockers such as *atenolol* block the heart from the effects of sympathetic stimulation, and this helps to reduce the heart's workload.

- Calcium channel blockers such as *diltiazem* vasodilate arterioles, slow the heart rate and reduce the force of contraction. All of these actions result in a reduction in the heart's workload.

- Potassium channel openers such as *nicorandil* act as vasodilators to reduce blood pressure, and they also have a nitrate-like action, dilating the coronary arteries.

- Funny channel blockers such as *ivabradine* slow the heart and reduce its oxygen demand.

Lipid-regulating drugs

The regulation of lipid metabolism

Cholesterol is a major constituent of the atherosclerotic plaques that develop in the coronary arteries. It is a lipid that is obtained from animal fats in the diet but can also be synthesised in the liver. The body needs a regular supply of cholesterol as it is important for the structural stability of cell membranes and forms the raw material for the manufacture of steroid hormones and vitamin D. It is also a component of bile produced by the liver.

Cholesterol is transported in the blood in small water-soluble spheres called **lipoproteins**. Being a lipid, cholesterol will not mix readily with blood which is watery in nature. In the centre of a lipoprotein sphere, however, the cholesterol is isolated from the blood by the phospholipid shell. This clever arrangement allows the lipoprotein sphere to dissolve in blood (Figure 4.11).

There are two clinically relevant types of lipoprotein - **high-density lipoprotein** (HDL) and **low-density lipoprotein** (LDL). The density of the two lipoproteins refers to the relative amounts of protein in the spheres but essentially it is the different roles that interest us. HDL scavenges cholesterol from tissues, removing it to the liver where it is stored, metabolised or incorporated into bile. LDL has a different role, including the transport of cholesterol from the liver to the tissues. Most importantly, it is LDL that is chemically modified and taken into developing atheromata by macrophages. Here it forms part of the developing atherosclerotic plaques.

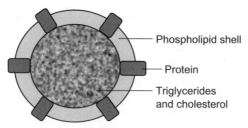

Phospholipid shell

Protein

Triglycerides and cholesterol

Figure 4.11 A lipoprotein sphere consisting of a phospholipid and protein shell isolating triglycerides and cholesterol from the watery environment of the blood.

The ratio between HDL and LDL is important. Generally, high levels of HDL and low levels of LDL are best for cardiovascular health. Lifestyle factors such as lack of exercise, high cholesterol diet and smoking can adversely affect the HDL : LDL ratio, decreasing HDL or increasing LDL levels.

> **KEY FACT**
>
> For **cardiovascular health**, it is important to reduce LDL and maximise HDL cholesterol.

Ideally, cholesterol levels should be controlled by diet, exercise and abstinence from harmful habits such as smoking and drinking too much alcohol. In reality, patients are often reluctant to change their lifestyle and for those at high risk from cardiovascular disease, pharmacological intervention can help to regulate cholesterol levels. The recommended UK values for cholesterol are as follows:

Recommended cholesterol values from NHS Direct

Total cholesterol	5.0 mmol/l* or lower
LDL (bad) cholesterol	3.0 mmol/l or lower
HDL (good) cholesterol	1.3 mmol/l or higher

* millimoles per litre (see below)

A BRIEF EXPLANATION of moles and molarity

Chemists measure quantities in moles, and 1 mole of a substance is about 6×10^{23} atoms. Molarity is the number of moles per litre of solution and 1 mole of a substance dissolved in 1 litre of water would be a 1 molar solution. The mole represents rather a lot of atoms so in biological chemistry you will generally find the millimole (mmol) rather than the mole. One millimole is one thousandth of a mole. Put simply, the greater the molarity, the more of a substance there is in a solution.

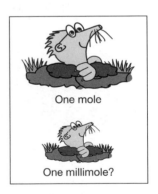

One mole

One millimole?

Drugs used to lower lipids: statins

The most commonly prescribed drugs used to lower serum cholesterol for the prevention and management of cardiovascular disease are statins. There are a few other drugs such as anion-exchange resins and fibrates but statins are by far the most popular. Examples of this group include *atorvastatin, fluvastatin, pravastatin, rosuvastatin* and *simvastatin*.

You might think that simply cutting down on fats in the diet would reduce cholesterol levels sufficiently but unfortunately, when cholesterol intake is reduced, the body can respond by manufacturing cholesterol in the liver. This can result in elevated serum cholesterol despite a reduction in dietary intake. Remember that cholesterol is a useful substance as well as a potentially harmful one so when levels fall then the body responds by making more of it.

KEY FACT

Reducing **cholesterol** intake may not be enough to control levels because the liver sometimes responds by synthesising more cholesterol.

Statins are inhibitors of the enzyme **3-hydroxy-3-methylglutaryl-Coenzyme A reductase**, usually (for obvious reasons) shortened to **HMG CoA reductase**. This enzyme takes part in a reaction in the pathway that produces cholesterol in the **hepatocytes** (liver cells) – Figures 4.12a and 4.12b. Because the liver needs cholesterol to make bile, when production is blocked by a statin, the hepatocytes pull more LDL cholesterol from the blood and this reduces circulating LDL and so reduces the risk of cardiovascular disease. Naturally statins need to be used in conjunction with a reduction in dietary intake of cholesterol, together with changes in lifestyle to ensure a healthy HDL : LDL ratio.

IN PRACTICE

Statins are generally taken in the evening because the liver is most active in the production of cholesterol at night.

Bile is the alkaline, detergent-like substance produced by the liver and secreted into the duodenum via the bile duct. Its main function is the emulsification of lipids that enables their digestion.

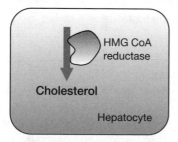

Figure 4.12a The hepatic enzyme HMG CoA reductase is involved in the production of cholesterol.

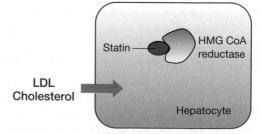

Figure 4.12b Statins block the action of HMG CoA reductase, inhibiting the production of cholesterol so hepatocytes import LDL cholesterol from the blood.

A QUICK RECAP on lipid-regulating drugs – statins

- Cholesterol is a lipid that is essential for the proper functioning of the body but it is also a key component of atherosclerotic plaques.

- We obtain cholesterol from our diet but it can also be synthesised by the liver.

- Cholesterol is transported in the blood in lipoprotein spheres. Two types are clinically important – high-density lipoprotein (HDL) and low-density lipoprotein (LDL).

- Ideally, LDL levels should be minimised and HDL levels maximised for good cardiovascular health.

- A sensible diet, abstaining from smoking and taking plenty of exercise helps regulate cholesterol levels.

- Statins inhibit HMG CoA reductase, a liver enzyme involved in the synthesis of cholesterol. A reduction in intracellular cholesterol also stimulates the hepatocytes to absorb LDL cholesterol from the blood.

Anticoagulant drugs

Let's start with the basics: what is clotting?

When someone gets injured it is important that blood loss is minimised otherwise they may eventually lose so much blood that they go into **shock**, a state where blood pressure falls to the point where tissues are not supplied with sufficient oxygen. Animals have therefore evolved a mechanism that responds to injury involving damage to blood vessels by converting the blood in the area of damage from its normal fluid form into a solid clot. This staunches the flow of blood and prevents further blood loss. Having dealt with the immediate emergency, further mechanisms are then initiated by the body to make more permanent repairs to the injured area in a process called **wound resolution**.

In most situations, clotting is a desirable process that prevents a loss of blood from a wound but in the case of the coronary arteries the formation of a clot on a ruptured plaque can be disastrous because it can cut off the blood supply to the heart muscle which could then die from lack of oxygen. In this chapter we will examine the process more closely and find out what drugs there are available to keep the blood flowing in the coronary arteries.

DID YOU KNOW ... that there is a sound reason for sucking your thumb when you have a small cut? Saliva contains an enzyme called lysozyme that attacks and destroys bacteria and so prevents your injury becoming infected.

What is a clot?

The blood clot itself is composed of three elements – **platelets**, **fibrin** and red blood cells. The platelets are small cell fragments that have the ability to bind to

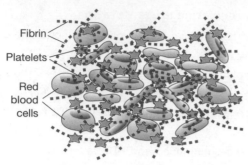

Fibrin

Platelets

Red blood cells

Figure 4.13 Blood clot showing the platelets, fibrin and red blood cells.

fibrin, a filament-like protein which forms a web-like structure that traps red blood cells and forms a clot. You can think of it as a fishing net, the platelets being the knots that tie the fibrin strands together (Figure 4.13).

Overview of clotting

Clotting, like most things in the body, is quite complex but can be understood more easily if we divide it into two key processes:

- **Activation of platelets** – these small cell-like structures are key players in the formation of a blood clot. Without them a clot will not form (a fact exploited by the many antiplatelet drugs).

- **Conversion of fibrinogen into fibrin** – fibrin is a thread-like protein that, together with platelets, forms a web that traps red blood cells. This is another process targeted by anticlotting drugs.

Part 1 of the clotting process: the activation of platelets

Platelets (also called **thrombocytes**) circulate in the blood and are key players in the clotting process. Produced primarily in the bone marrow, they are disc shaped cell fragments without a nucleus and 3-4 µm diameter. Around 300 million are found in each millilitre of blood with an average life of around ten days. Platelets are generally inactive as they circulate in the blood until they come into contact with proteins such as **collagen** in the wall of a damaged blood vessel. This activates the platelets which change their shape from smooth to spiky and they also produce receptors on their cell membrane. These receptors, designated **GPIIb/IIIa receptors**, bind to circulating fibrin, making the web that entraps red blood cells and forms the clot (Figure 4.14).

The mechanisms involved in the activation of platelets needs to be explained briefly in order that you can understand the action of two key anticlotting drugs, *aspirin* and *clopidogrel*. In response to tissue damage, platelets become activated and produce two chemicals, **thromboxane A_2** (TXA_2) and **adenosine diphosphate** (ADP) that cause the platelets to increase the production of GPIIb/IIIa receptors and display them on their cell surface where they can bind to fibrin.

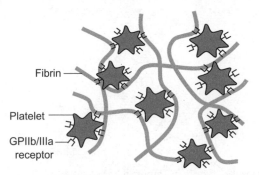

Figure 4.14 Activated platelets bind to fibrin by their GPIIb/IIIa receptors.

ANOTHER WAY TO PICTURE THIS

Imagine the platelets as children in a cold playground so they have their hands (receptors) in their pockets. On the floor are lots of skipping ropes (fibrin) and when the teacher blows a whistle all the children take their hands out of their pockets and grab hold of any two skipping ropes forming a kind of net. Hold onto this picture because we will come back to it later when discussing antiplatelet drugs.

Part 2 of the clotting process: the conversion of fibrinogen into fibrin

We have seen how the platelets are activated and now we will look at the second important process in the formation of a blood clot, the conversion of fibrinogen into fibrin. In the blood, fibrin circulates as an inactive soluble protein called fibrinogen. Because it is soluble when dissolved in the blood, fibrinogen will not interact with the platelets because the GPIIb/IIIa receptors cannot bind to it. Imagine trying to grab hold of jelly – that's like platelets trying to bind to fibrinogen. However, when fibrinogen is converted into fibrin it becomes insoluble and visible and can be seen through a high power electron microscope as tiny, cotton-like threads. In this form, the platelet GPIIb/IIIa receptors bind eagerly to fibrin and form the web-like structure that traps the red blood cells and forms the blood clot.

The clotting process looks pretty complex.

Yes, it is quite complex but you really need to know how the clotting process works in order to understand the action of common anti-clotting drugs such as *aspirin*, *clopidogrel*, *heparin* and *warfarin*.

Circulating in the blood are a family of clotting proteins (also known as clotting factors), most of which are identified simply by Roman numerals. Fibrinogen itself is one of these proteins and is designated Factor I. Fibrinogen is converted into fibrin (Factor Ia) as the result of a cascade of enzymic reactions involving these clotting factors.

The clotting cascade is triggered by either blood coming into contact with damaged tissue or exposed collagen. This causes the activation of clotting factors VIII or XII, each of which activates another clotting factor in the cascade and this activates the next factor and so on. In Figure 4.15 you will note that the factors

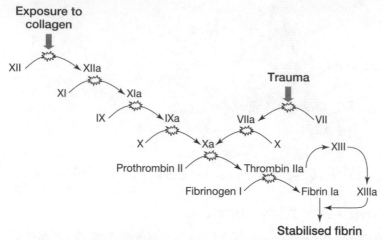

Figure 4.15 The clotting cascade (simplified). Injury or exposure of the blood to the connective tissue collagen causes a series of reactions in the blood that result in the formation of stabilised fibrin, a key component of blood clots.

when activated take the suffix 'a' ('a' stands for activated). Eventually an enzyme called **prothrombin** (Factor II) is converted to its active form of **thrombin** (Factor IIa). Thrombin is of key importance because it converts soluble fibrinogen into stabilised insoluble fibrin with the help of Factor VIIIa. In its stable, insoluble form, fibrin and platelets together form the web-like structure that traps blood cells and makes the blood clot.

Drugs used to prevent clotting

Individuals who have coronary artery disease are at greater risk of clots forming and blocking their coronary arteries, resulting in ischaemia and infarction. The aim of anticoagulant therapy therefore is to interfere with the clotting process and so reduce the chances of clots forming, especially in the coronary arteries. As we have seen, there are two key processes involved in the clotting process – the activation of platelets and the conversion of fibrinogen into fibrin. Drugs used to inhibit clotting can also be broadly divided into two groups: antiplatelet drugs and drugs targeting the clotting cascade.

> **KEY FACT**
>
> **Anticlotting drugs** work either by inhibiting the activity of platelets or by inhibiting the clotting cascade that converts fibrinogen into fibrin.

Anticoagulant drugs group 1: antiplatelet drugs

There are many drugs used to inhibit the activation of platelets but the two that you are most likely to encounter are *aspirin* and *clopidogrel*. Both of these drugs act on platelets and prevent them from expressing the GPIIb/IIIa receptors that bind to fibrin, producing the web-like structure that traps red blood cells and forms the blood clot. Other antiplatelet drugs such as **dipyridamole**, **tirofiban**, **eptifibatide** and **abciximab** tend to be used only in specialist cardiology units for patients at high risk of myocardial infarction or undergoing surgical procedures such as percutaneous coronary intervention (see Section 4.2 towards the beginning of this chapter).

Aspirin is one of our oldest non-steroidal anti-inflammatory drugs (NSAIDs) and although used less often these days as an analgesic for pain relief, it has found a new role as an antiplatelet drug for the prevention of myocardial infarction. It is also used to prevent a **stroke** which involves a similar pathology to coronary artery disease but in this case the atherosclerotic plaques form in the **carotid arteries** that supply the brain with oxygen. Rupture of a plaque in these arteries can cause a clot to develop that cuts off blood to the brain, sometimes causing permanent damage.

Aspirin or **acetylsalicylic acid** works by inhibiting the production of a locally acting chemical called **thromboxane A$_2$** (TXA$_2$) – one of the prostaglandin family of mediators that are produced in inflammation. We will meet prostaglandins again in Chapter 7. Activated platelets produce thromboxane, which increases the production of GPIIb/IIIa receptors that bind to fibrin and form the blood clot as described earlier. TXA$_2$ is produced from **arachidonic acid** by an enzyme called **cyclo-oxygenase 1** (COX-1) (see Chapter 7). *Aspirin* irreversibly binds to COX-1, inhibiting its action and so preventing platelets making thromboxane and expressing their receptors (Figure 4.16). Without receptors, platelets cannot bind to fibrin and the clot cannot form.

> **Stroke** is a serious disturbance in the blood supply to the brain caused by the formation of a blood clot or haemorrhage in the arteries that supply the brain.

As the inhibition of COX-1 is irreversible it means that the platelet cannot produce any more GPIIb/IIIa receptors. However, platelets only have a life of around 10 days so the clotting function is restored as new platelets are produced.

> **DID YOU KNOW...** that *aspirin* was originally obtained from willow bark? Willow is *Salix* in Latin and its name can still be traced in the chemical name of *aspirin* – acetylsalicylic acid.

Clopidogrel also works by inhibiting the production of GPIIb/IIIa receptors on platelets but by a different mechanism to aspirin. Adenosine diphosphate (ADP) is a mediator produced during platelet activation that stimulates the production of GPIIb/IIIa receptors by binding to and stimulating ADP receptors on the surface of the platelets (Figure 4.19). *Clopidogrel* is an ADP antagonist that

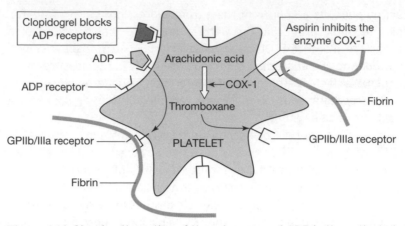

Figure 4.16 Showing the action of thromboxane and ADP in the activated platelet. Both mediators increase the expression of GPIIb/IIIa receptors and promote the clotting process. *Aspirin* and *clopidogrel* inhibit both of these mediators and so discourage clotting.

blocks ADP receptors, preventing ADP binding and so inhibiting the expression of GPIIb/IIIa receptors.

ANOTHER WAY TO PICTURE THIS

Remember that we compared platelets to children in a playground? As it's cold, they have their hands (receptors) in their pockets. *Aspirin* and *clopidogrel* induce the children to keep their hands firmly in their pockets to prevent them grasping the skipping ropes (fibrin) that forms the web-like net (clot).

Side-effects Aspirin can cause gastro-intestinal haemorrhage. Prostaglandins have a protective effect on the gastric mucosa and their production is inhibited by aspirin. *Aspirin* (and other NSAIDs) can also induce asthma (see 'In practice' below). *Clopidogrel* can cause the usual gastric upsets and may also lead to bleeding disorders. See the current BNF for a full list of side-effects of both drugs.

IN PRACTICE

It is estimated that around 10% of asthma sufferers are sensitive to *aspirin* and other non-steroidal anti-inflammatory drugs (NSAIDs). They can induce an asthma attack, often accompanied by symptoms of runny nose, sneezing and facial flushing. The mechanism is uncertain but NSAIDs may increase the production of **leukotrienes**, mediators implicated in asthma.

Anticoagulant drugs group 2: drugs acting on the clotting cascade

This group of drugs includes **heparins** and *warfarin* as well as some of the less-well-known anticoagulants such as the **hirudins** and *fondaparinux*. As these last two are unlikely to be encountered outside of specialist surgical settings, we will only mention them in passing.

Heparins are mainly used in hospitals and are prescribed primarily to prevent deep-vein thrombosis and pulmonary embolism in patients undergoing surgery. They are also used extensively in coronary care for patients with unstable angina and to prevent clots forming after cardiac interventions. *Heparin* is unsuitable for oral administration and is therefore delivered either by intravenous infusion or by subcutaneous injection. There are two forms of *heparin* in current use, the original **unfractionated** *heparin* and the more recently introduced **low molecular weight** *heparin* (LMW heparin). Examples of LMW heparins include *bemiparin*, *dalteparin*, *enoxaparin* and *tinzaparin*. Heparins inhibit clotting by activating a protein called **antithrombin**, part of the body's own anticlotting mechanism. Antithrombin, as the name implies, inactivates thrombin but also inhibits various other clotting factors (Figure 4.17). Unfractionated *heparin* and *LMW heparin* effectively do the same task in activating antithrombin, but there are small differences in which of the other clotting factors they inhibit.

IN PRACTICE

The clots that form in the veins are subtly different from those that form in the arteries. Arterial clots generally form in response to vascular injury and this activates platelets so these clots are said to be platelet rich. Venous thrombi, on the other hand, more often form due to inadequate blood flow and so are fibrin rich and platelet poor. This is why drugs such as *heparin* and *warfarin* rather than antiplatelet drugs are used to prevent deep vein thrombosis.

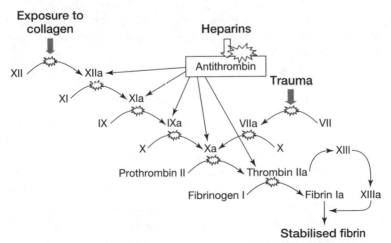

Figure 4.17 Heparins activate the natural anticlotting protein antithrombin that in turn deactivates various clotting factors as shown in the diagram. The clotting cascade is halted, preventing the formation of stabilised fibrin, a key component of blood clots.

Side-effects As with all anticoagulants, *heparin* can cause unwanted bleeding and it can also result in heparin-induced **thrombocytopenia** (low platelet levels).

> ## CASE STUDY
>
> Betty has been admitted for a hip replacement and with the prospect of her remaining immobile for several weeks there is the risk of DVT developing. Apart from a suspected peptic ulcer, Betty is otherwise in reasonable health. Would you advise *aspirin* to prevent DVT - or perhaps some other anti-clotting drug?

Comment on case study Aspirin should not be given to anyone with a peptic ulcer, as there is a strong risk of causing a **gastro-intestinal** (GI) bleed. All anticoagulant drugs have the potential to cause problems in patients at risk from bleeding. Non-pharmacological solutions such as thromboembolism deterrent (TED) stockings may be a better option.

Warfarin is an oral anticoagulant used for prevention of deep vein thrombosis (DVT), pulmonary embolism, atrial fibrillation and after the surgical insertion of prosthetic heart valves.

Warfarin acts in the liver to prevent the production of clotting Factors II, VII, IX and X. Being similar in structure to vitamin K, it binds to and inhibits the enzyme vitamin K reductase, a key enzyme in the production of clotting factors. As the number of clotting factors in the blood diminishes, so does the body's ability to form sufficient fibrin to make structurally stable clots. The most common side-effect with *warfarin* is unwanted bleeding.

> ## IN PRACTICE
>
> The anticoagulant effects of *warfarin* take 48-72 hours to develop fully. This is because *warfarin* inhibits the synthesis of new clotting factors but does not affect those already in circulation.

Anticoagulant drugs group 3: fibrinolytic drugs

So far we have seen how both groups of anticlotting drugs, antiplatelet and coagulation cascade inhibitors can prevent clots from forming in the arteries and veins. We will now examine drugs that can be used in emergency situations where a patient is having a myocardial infarction caused by a blood clot that has formed in the coronary arteries. We now need powerful drugs that will break down and disperse a blood clot, thus restoring blood and life-giving oxygen to heart tissue. These drugs are called **fibrinolytic** or **thrombolytic** drugs because they **lyse** (break down) fibrin and consequently the structural integrity of the thrombus collapses. These drugs include *alteplase, reteplase, streptokinase* and *tenecteplase*.

All of these drugs act by stimulating **plasmin,** the body's own clot-busting enzyme that breaks down fibrin. Plasmin is formed from its inactive form **plasminogen** that

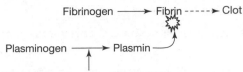

Figure 4.18 Showing how plasminogen is converted into its clot-destroying form of plasmin by tissue plasmin activator (t-PA).

becomes incorporated into the clot as it forms. The body needs to ensure that when a wound has healed the clot will dissolve as part of the repair process. Plasminogen is eventually converted into plasmin by a protein called **tissue plasminogen activator** (t-PA) – Figure 4.18. Fibrinolytic drugs are similar in structure to t-PA and so produce activated plasmin that breaks down fibrin and dissolves the clot.

Streptokinase is a bacterial enzyme derived from **β-haemolytic streptococci**. As a foreign, bacterial protein it can trigger an immunological reaction and is therefore not used beyond four days after its first use. After that period, antibodies produced in response to the initial administration will attack and neutralise the drug.

Alteplase, *tenecteplase* and *reteplase* are **recombinant** tissue plasminogen activators (rt-PA) that act by the same mechanism as *streptokinase* but are more specific for clot-bound plasminogen and also, being non-bacterial in origin, do not elicit the same immune response as *streptokinase*. Recombinant technology involves genetic manipulation, removing a gene from one organism and splicing it into another, generally a bacterium or yeast, in order to produce significant quantities of a protein – in this case, tissue plasminogen activator.

> **CASE STUDY**
>
> Sam, an agricultural worker collapses at work, complaining of shortness of breath and severe 'indigestion' like pain that is spreading up his left side. An ambulance arrives within 20 minutes and the paramedics perform an electrocardiogram (ECG) on Sam. After consulting with the hospital they decide to administer 10,000 units of *tenecteplase* by intravenous (IV) injection. What is happening to Sam?

Comment on case study Sam has the classic symptoms of a myocardial infarction or heart attack. The ECG would show subtle changes in the heart's electrical activity that are signs of a MI. Because Sam works in the countryside he may be some distance from a hospital, therefore to restore the blood supply to his heart muscle, thrombolysis will be performed by the paramedics. Sam's prospects for survival and recovery are better with early treatment.

> **Antibodies**, or immunoglobulins, are potent immune proteins produced by B-lymphocytes in the lymph nodes. Released into the bloodstream they attach themselves to invading **pathogens** and mark them for destruction by white blood cells.

A QUICK RECAP on drugs used to prevent clotting

- Clotting is the body's emergency repair system that prevents excessive blood loss after injury.

- Clots consist of fibrin strands cross-linked by platelets. This forms a mesh-like structure that traps red blood cells.

- Anticlotting drugs can be divided into two types – drugs acting on platelets and drugs acting on the coagulation cascade.

- Antiplatelet drugs such as *aspirin* and *clopidogrel* inhibit platelets from expressing GPIIb/IIIa receptors so they cannot bind to fibrin.

- Drugs such as *heparin* that act on the coagulation cascade interfere with the clotting cascade and so prevent fibrinogen being converted into fibrin.

- Drugs such as *warfarin* that act on the coagulation cascade inhibit an enzyme in the liver responsible for producing circulating clotting factors. As circulating levels of these factors diminish, so does the blood's ability to form clots.

- In emergencies, such as a heart attack, thrombolytic drugs such as *streptokinase* convert plasminogen into plasmin – an enzyme that breaks down blood clots.

Arrhythmias and anti-arrhythmic drugs

The use of drugs to control arrhythmias (abnormal heart rhythms) is a very specialised area and it is beyond the scope of this introductory book to explain the action of these drugs in any great detail. However, some anti-arrhythmic drugs such as *amiodarone, verapamil, digoxin* and β-blockers are regularly pre-scribed to people with heart problems, so it is worth discussing them briefly to ensure that you are at least familiar with their names.

If you place your fingers half way down your rib cage, just to the left of your **sternum** (breast bone), you should feel the steady, rhythmic beating of your heart. This is called **sinus rhythm** and is set by the heart's main pacemaker, the **sino-atrial (SA) node**, located in the front wall of the right atrium. The SA node generates a regular impulse which spreads across the heart muscle caus-ing it to contract and force blood out of the atria and ventricles respectively. The SA node rate is governed by efferent nerves from the parasympathetic and sympathetic divisions of the autonomic system. Normally the parasympathetic division dominates at rest, keeping the heart rate at its resting level, typically between 65 and 75 beats per minute. During exercise or stress, the sympathetic division becomes dominant and the rate increases, causing the heart to pump more oxygenated blood around the body.

There are many types and many causes of cardiac arrhythmias that require specialist diagnosis, usually with the aid of an **electrocardiogram** (ECG), a device that measures electrical activity in the heart and displays that activity as a series of traces on a graph. This enables clinicians to determine the location and nature of any abnormalities in heart function.

Some arrhythmias are defined by an abnormal heart rate – either **tachycardia** (excessively fast rate) or **bradycardia** (excessively slow rate). Tachycardia may be caused by pain, stress, fever, shock or by drugs such as *salbutamol*. Hypothermia can cause bradycardia as can drugs such as *digoxin* and β-blockers. Some arrhythmias are the result of damage to the heart's internal conduction system, often caused by heart attacks that can result in cells outside the SA node starting to act as pacemakers and sending abnormal signals across the myocardium. Sometimes, the impulse that spreads across the heart muscle in one direction then turns back on itself and becomes a circular **re-entrant** rhythm. Whatever the cause of the arrhythmia, it will affect the normal pumping of the heart and clinical intervention is often needed to restore a normal rhythm.

Anti-arrhythmic drugs

Amiodarone is a drug commonly used to prevent arrhythmias although its mechanism of action is not fully understood. It is believed to block some of the K^+ and Na^+ (and possibly Ca^{2+}) channels on the heart's conduction tissue and muscle cells. This slows the wave of contraction with each heart beat, helping to produce a more stable rhythm. This drug has a propensity to cause many side-effects and with an average half-life of over 30 days, these side-effects are not easily reversible. Unusually, *amiodarone* contains iodine and having structural similarities to the thyroid hormone **thyroxine**, this can affect iodine metabolism, sometimes resulting in **hypothyroidism** (low levels of thyroxine) and, less frequently, in **hyperthyroidism** (high levels of thyroxine). Deposits in the cornea of the eye are common with long-term use as is the tendency for *amiodarone* to cause the skin to turn blue-grey when exposed to sunlight.

- *Verapamil*, discussed earlier in this chapter in its role as an anti-anginal drug, helps to prevent arrhythmias by blocking Ca^{2+} channels especially in the heart's conduction tissue, thus slowing the heart and helping in the treatment of tachycardias.

- *Digoxin* is a cardiac glycoside found in the purple foxglove *Digitalis purpurea*. It has a complex action that increases Ca^{2+} concentration in the myocytes which, in turn, increases the force of contraction of the myocardium. It also acts on the central nervous system, reinforcing parasympathetic activity and reducing heart rate.

- **β-blockers** are used for several cardiovascular problems including angina, hypertension and heart failure. Those used as anti-arrhythmics include *propranolol*, *atenolol*, *esmolol*, *metoprolol* and *sotalol*. The action of these drugs was discussed earlier in this chapter in the section on anti-anginal drugs, but essentially they block $β_1$ receptors on the heart from the effects of adrenaline and noradrenaline and this reduces heart rate and contractility. *Sotalol* appears also to have a broad spectrum of anti-arrhythmic activity similar to that of *amiodarone*.

A QUICK RECAP on arrhythmias and anti-arrhythmic drugs

- **Arrhythmias** (abnormal heart rhythms) can be caused by heart disease or as a side-effect of some drugs.

- The diagnosis and treatment of arrhythmias is complex and requires specialist clinical knowledge.

- Anti-arrhythmic drugs such as *amiodarone*, *verapamil* and β-blockers work by a variety of mechanisms but they all have an inhibitory action on the heart rate and slow the speed of contraction of the myocardium.

- *Digoxin* slows the heart rate and increases the force of contraction of the myocardium.

RUNNING WORDS

Here are some of the technical terms that were included in this chapter. Read through them one by one and tick them off when you are sure that you understand them.

Acetylsalicylic acid p. 99	Diastole p. 80	Lyse p. 102
Adenosine diphosphate p. 96	Electrocardiogram p. 104	Macrophages p. 82
Antithrombin p. 101	Fatty streaks p. 82	Myocardial infarction p. 82
Aorta p. 79	Fibrin p. 95	Myocardium p. 79
Apex p. 79	Fibrinolytic p. 102	Occluded p. 84
Arachidonic acid p. 99	Funny channel p. 91	Pathogens p. 103
Arteries p. 77	Gastro-intestinal p. 102	Percutaneous coronary interventions p. 85
Arterioles p. 78	GP11b/111a receptors p. 96	Plaques p. 82
Atheroma p. 82	Heart failure p. 84	Plasmin p. 102
Atheromata p. 82	Heparins p. 100	Plasminogen p. 102
Atherosclerosis p. 82	Hepatocytes p. 94	Platelets p. 95
Atria p. 79	High-density lipoprotein (HDL) p. 92	Prothrombin p. 98
Atrioventricular valve p. 79	HMG CoA reductase p. 94	Pulmonary arteries p. 79
β-haemolytic streptococci p. 103	Hyperthyroidism p. 105	Pulmonary system p. 77
Bradycardia p. 105	Hypothyroidism p. 105	Pulmonary veins p. 79
Capillaries p. 77	Infarct p. 84	Radiographic imaging p. 85
Carotid p. 82	Ischaemic p. 84	Recombinant p. 103
Catheter p. 85	Lactic acid p. 84	Re-entrant p. 105
Collagen p. 96	Leukotrienes p. 100	Referred pain p. 84
Coronary artery bypass graft p. 85	Lipoproteins p. 92	Semilunar valve p. 79
Coronary circulation p. 81	Low-density lipoprotein (LDL) p. 92	Shock p. 95
Cyclo-oxygenase 1 p. 99	Low molecular weight heparin p. 101	Sino-atrial node p. 104

REFERENCES AND FURTHER RECOMMENDED READING

All recommended websites are open access (but free registration is sometimes required).

UK Statistics Authority – http://www.statistics.gov.uk

Opie, L.H. and Gersh, B.J. (2008) *Drugs for the Heart* (7th edition). Saunders.

Student, B.M.J. – http://student.bmj.com/topics/clinical/cardiovascular_medicine.php

British Heart Foundation – http://www.bhf.org.uk/

Bandolier: cardiology – http://www.medicine.ox.ac.uk/bandolier/

Your turn to try

Now you have finished reading this chapter it is time to find out how much you have learned and remembered. No one pretends that pharmacology is the easiest of subjects to study so don't worry if you can't answer some of the questions and have to go back a few pages in Chapter 4 to reread a particular section – this is all part of the learning process.

The answers to these questions are at the end of the book on page 284.

1 List at least six functions of the circulatory system.

2 In which of the blood vessels does exchange between the blood and the cells takes place?

3 What is the name of the blood vessels that supply blood to the myocardium?

4 What is the main lipid found in atherosclerotic plaques?

5 Why may an artery that is partially blocked by a plaque result in angina pain?

6 GTN dilates the coronary arteries – why may this reduce angina pain?

7 What might be the consequence of a plaque rupturing in the coronary arteries?

8 Why would slowing the heart rate with a beta-blocker reduce angina pain?

9 What type of circulating lipoprotein is implicated in the formation of plaques?

10 Why may reducing dietary cholesterol not always result in a fall in blood cholesterol?

11 How does inhibiting HMG CoA reductase with a statin reduce blood cholesterol?

12 What are the three main components of a blood clot?

13 How does aspirin prevent clotting?

14 What is the key difference between the action of warfarin and heparins?

15 In what circumstances might a thrombolytic drug be used?

Answers to questions on page 75

1 Neither, it is in the middle of the chest.
2 From the heart.
3 Four chambers – two atria and two ventricles.
4 Arteries, capillaries and veins.
5 The coronary arteries.

Chapter 5

The cardiovascular system (2)

Hypertension and antihypertensive drugs

AIMS

By the time you have finished the chapter you will understand:

1 The **physiology** – how the body regulates blood pressure
2 The **pathology** – hypertension and its consequences
3 The **pharmacology** – action of the major antihypertensive drug groups

CONTENTS

The chapter contains some brief case studies and finishes off with some self-test questions to enable you to be certain that you have understood the physiology, pathology and pharmacology of this important area.

IN PRACTICE

Blood pressure is something that everyone in clinical practice needs to understand because almost everyone in clinical practice will need to measure blood pressure, perhaps the most common of clinical procedures, at some time in their professional career. The maintenance of a healthy blood pressure is essential for the efficient functioning of the body and problems occur if blood pressure deviates significantly from its healthy norm. If blood pressure falls then the patient can go into shock and this is a medical emergency that requires emergency action. A rise in blood pressure tends to be a long-term problem rather than an emergency but the consequences can be quite serious. Regardless of their pathology, it is likely that many of your adult patients will have high blood pressure and will be taking medication to reduce their blood pressure, so it is essential that you understand how both antihypertensive drugs and the body itself work to regulate blood pressure.

Introduction

High blood pressure or **hypertension** is a very common problem, especially in developed countries such as the UK where, by the age of 50, almost 25 per cent of the population are hypertensive. People who have sustained high blood pressure are at greater risk of developing diseases such as diabetes and heart problems, so it makes sense for them to take steps to reduce it. Ideally, a reduction in blood pressure should be achieved with changes in diet and exercise, but antihypertensive drugs are an alternative for the many people who find it difficult to change their lifestyle. There are many different drugs with a wide variety of actions and this chapter examines them in detail.

This chapter follows a format that will be becoming familiar to you. Firstly, we make sure that we understand the physiology – the nature of blood pressure and how the body maintains that blood pressure. Secondly, we need to understand the pathology of hypertension, what causes it and its consequences. Finally we put this knowledge to good use when we explore the pharmacology, how the main groups of antihypertensive drugs work to lower blood pressure. Case studies and clinical scenarios will help to reinforce your understanding of this subject.

WHERE ARE WE STARTING FROM?

Before you start this chapter you need to have read (and remembered) the basics of circulatory physiology that we covered in Chapter 4. Let's see how much you have learned . . .

1 Which blood vessel carries blood from the heart to major organs such as the kidneys and liver?

_____

2 Which side of the heart (left or right) pumps blood to the lungs?

_____

3 When blood returns to the heart from the veins, does it first enter the atria or the ventricles?

_____

4 Which is the highest pressure in the blood vessels – systole or diastole?

_____

5 Do the pulmonary veins carry oxygenated or deoxygenated blood?

_____

6 Is the vena-cava a vein or an artery?

_____

Answers are at the end of the chapter on page 136.

Good, we will assume that you answered all or most of the answers correctly and that you know the basic structures and functions of the circulatory system. We can now get down to learning about blood pressure, hypertension and the anti-hypertensive drugs. If you struggled with these questions, perhaps you should reread the section in Chapter 4 that explains the basics of circulatory physiology.

5.1 The physiology of blood pressure

Let's start with the basics: what is blood pressure?

When we talk about blood pressure, we are generally referring to the pressure of blood in systemic arteries such as the aorta. As we saw in Chapter 4, the systemic arteries are those that carry blood from the left side of the heart, via the aorta, to the organs and tissues of the body. These organs include the brain, liver, kidneys and digestive system and tissues such as the muscles and skin. Naturally, the blood is also under pressure in the pulmonary arteries carrying blood from the right

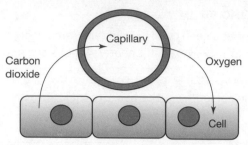

Figure 5.1 Capillaries, the smallest of our blood vessels, supply cells with oxygen and remove carbon dioxide.

side of the heart to the lungs, but this pressure is much lower and not as easy to measure because the pulmonary arteries lie deep within the **thoracic cavity**.

Arterial pressure is important to the well-being of the body because it is this pressure that causes oxygenated blood from the lungs to flow to the cells of the organs and tissues. This pressure pushes the blood through the arteries and into the tiny capillaries of the body where gas exchange takes place between the blood and the cells. These capillaries permeate every cubic millimetre of the body and are essential for the health of our cells. A constant supply of fresh blood is required to supply cells with their oxygen and nutrients and take away wastes such as the gas, carbon dioxide (Figure 5.1). If pressure falls and the blood moves more slowly through the capillaries, then cells do not get enough oxygen and cannot get rid of their carbon dioxide.

Understanding arterial blood pressure

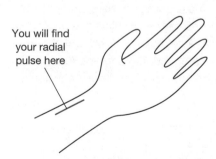

Figure 5.2 How to find your radial pulse.

Arterial pressure is **pulsatile** in nature in that it fluctuates between a high pressure and a low pressure. The maximum pressure of blood on the arterial walls is the **systolic** pressure and the lowest pressure is the **diastolic**. Some systemic arteries appear near the surface of the body and pressure changes in these arteries can be measured relatively easily with the familiar **sphygmomanometer**, generally shortened to 'sphyg'. Place the tips of your first and second finger in the groove just below the end of your **radius** bone and you will experience the systolic expansion of the arteries as a pulse in the **radial artery** just under the skin (Figure 5.2).

Sphygmomanometer is a device for measuring systemic arterial blood pressure. An inflatable fabric cuff wrapped round the upper arm detects systolic and diastolic pressures. Results are displayed digitally (although some mercury column sphygs are still in use).

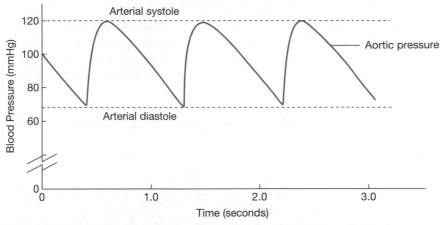

Figure 5.3 Typical blood pressures in a systemic artery such as the aorta.

The heart beats around 70 times each minute and with each beat the ventricles contract and force blood into the arteries. The elastic walls of the arteries stretch as the pressure increases to maximum systolic pressure. Then, when the heart goes into its diastolic phase and relaxes, their elastic walls steadily recoil, continuing to push the blood through the millions of tiny arterioles and capillaries.

Figure 5.3 is a simplified graph of fluctuations in blood pressure in a systemic artery such as the aorta. Note that there is always a minimum pressure in the arteries of (typically) 70-80 mmHg. Because there is always this pressure in the arteries, there is always a constant flow, pushing blood through the arterioles and capillaries.

The rapid rise in pressure seen in Figure 5.3 is caused by the ventricles contracting, forcing blood into the arteries – this is systole. As the heart relaxes to fill with blood again, the pressure in the arteries falls as the blood is pushed through the arterioles and capillaries – this is diastole.

> **KEY FACT**
>
> The blood pressure in the arteries fluctuates with each heart beat between systole (maximum pressure) and diastole (minimum pressure).

The control of arterial blood pressure

It is very important that systemic arterial blood pressure is maintained sufficiently high to drive the blood through the millions of capillaries to provide nutrient supply, gas exchange and waste removal from the cells of the body's tissues, but not so high that it ruptures the small blood vessels or places undue strain on the heart.

Maintaining blood pressure is very important and is subject to constant monitoring and adjustment by the body to make sure that it never falls so low as to compromise the blood supply to essential organs such as the brain.

Blood pressure is maintained in the short term by the complex interaction of **systemic vascular resistance** (SVR) and **cardiac output** (CO). Longer-term regulation also calls for adjustment to blood volume. We are going to look at the long-term and short-term control of blood pressure because we will need to understand them when we later examine the action of antihypertensive drugs.

The short-term regulation of blood pressure

> **KEY FACT**
>
> The short-term regulation of blood pressure is largely determined by two factors – cardiac output and systemic vascular resistance.

The following facts are very important so we will state them separately:

1 **Cardiac output** (CO) is the amount of blood pumped by the heart each minute.
2 Cardiac output is determined by two factors:
   (a) **Heart rate** (HR) – the rate at which the heart beats;
   (b) **Stroke volume** (SV) – the amount of blood pumped by the ventricle each beat.
3 **Systemic vascular resistance** (SVR) is the resistance to blood flow as determined by peripheral blood vessel diameter in the systemic circulation.

ANOTHER WAY TO PICTURE THIS

Imagine the arterial system like a long, thin balloon with a small hole in the far end. To maintain pressure in the balloon you have to blow regularly into one end (cardiac output) and restrict the amount of air coming out of the hole at the other end (systemic vascular resistance).

Blood viscosity and the total length of blood vessels also contribute to systemic vascular resistance, but they remain relatively static in the short term so SVR is largely determined by the diameter of the smallest of arteries, the arterioles.

We can best express the relationship of the factors that determine blood pressure by a simple formula:

$$BP = CO \times SVR$$
(Blood pressure = Cardiac output × Systemic vascular resistance)

Cardiac output is expressed by another simple formula:

$$CO = HR \times SV$$
(Cardiac output = Heart rate × Stroke volume)

Do I really need to learn this formula?

YES (sorry to shout) – you most certainly do! You don't need to learn many formulae to study basic physiology but this one is very important – if not *the* most important. So it is worth spending a few minutes working through this section to make sure you understand it.

If formulae are a bit of a mystery to you then just substitute some values instead of the words. For example, a typical heart rate might be 70 beats per minute (bpm) and typical stroke volume 70 millilitres (ml) of blood.

$$\text{Cardiac output} = 70 \text{ bpm} \times 70 \text{ ml}$$

This gives us a typical cardiac output of 4900 millilitres, nearly 5 litres of blood pumped each minute. Because the formula indicates that the figure on the left side of the equal sign is determined by the product of everything on the right of the equal sign, this means if you change either of the two figures on the right side then the figure on the left side changes. For example, if the individual started to exercise, then heart rate and stroke volume might both increase as follows:

$$\text{Cardiac output} = 100 \text{ bpm} \times 85 \text{ ml}$$

This means that cardiac output increases to 8500 millilitres of blood pumped each minute. Similarly, if anything on the right side of the formula decreases, then the figure on the left side decreases. Perhaps the individual has an accident causing loss of blood which causes a reduction in stroke volume as follows:

$$\text{Cardiac output} = 70 \text{ bpm} \times 50 \text{ ml}$$

In this case, cardiac output falls to 3500 millilitres of blood pumped each minute.
Going back to our blood pressure formula . . .

$$BP = CO \times SVR$$

This just indicates that blood pressure (BP) is equal to the product of cardiac output (CO) and systemic vascular resistance (SVR). It also indicates that if either CO or SVR increase, then BP will increase. On the other hand, if either CO or SVR decrease, then BP will decrease. This gives us a clue as to how the body will respond to changes in blood pressure.

KEY FACT

If either CO or SVR increase then BP will increase. If either CO or SVR decrease then BP will decrease.

First we need to understand the mechanisms that the body has at its disposal to regulate blood pressure.

REALITY CHECK

The blood pressure formula is very important if you are to understand how the body regulates BP - and also how antihypertensive drugs work. Without looking at the book, can you write down the formula and explain how the various factors interact to the control of blood pressure?

Systemic vascular resistance

Systemic vascular resistance is defined as the combined resistance of the peripheral arterioles of the systemic circulation. Arterioles are surrounded by bands of smooth muscle and when these collectively contract, the diameter of the lumen of the vessel decreases and this increases resistance.

ANOTHER WAY TO PICTURE THIS

Imagine a crowd of football fans leaving through the stadium gates at the end of the game. If someone were to partially close some of the gates, pressure in the jostling crowd would increase. Vasoconstriction has the same effect, making it harder for the blood to flow through the arterioles and so increasing the pressure in the arteries.

Arterioles are controlled by both the nervous system and chemical messengers released into the blood as a response to changes (generally falls) in blood pressure. Each arteriole is connected to the central nervous system by nerves from the sympathetic division of the autonomic nervous system. The autonomic nervous system is formed from groups of nerves originating in the central nervous system that maintain homeostasis - the steady state of the internal environment. When blood pressure drops, the sympathetic division is activated to restore pressure to within normal values. Sympathetic nerves connected to arterioles cause each arteriole to contract, resulting in an increase in systemic vascular resistance (Figure 5.4).

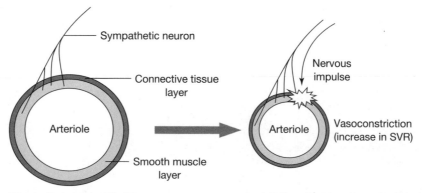

Figure 5.4 Sympathetic nerves cause vasoconstriction that increases systemic vascular resistance (SVR).

Table 5.1 The chemical messengers that cause contraction of smooth muscle cells on the peripheral arterioles

Chemical messenger	Source of messenger	Target receptor on smooth muscle cell	Action on smooth muscle cell
Noradrenaline	Sympathetic neurons	α_1 adrenergic receptor	Contraction
Adrenaline	Adrenal gland	α_1 adrenergic receptor	Contraction
Angiotensin II	Circulating	Angiotensin-II receptor	Contraction
ADH-vasopressin	Posterior pituitary	ADH-vasopressin receptor	Contraction

To understand how sympathetic stimulation results in vasoconstriction of the arterioles, we need to examine their structure, in particular the bands of tiny smooth muscle cells that lie in layers around the arterioles. Sympathetic stimulation causes these cells to contract in unison which, in turn, causes the arteriole to contract, reducing its diameter and increasing systemic vascular resistance. These muscle cells respond to the sympathetic neurotransmitter noradrenaline plus a variety of chemical messengers that circulate in the blood. Each of these chemical messengers has its own receptor on the smooth muscle cells that initiates contraction (Table 5.1 and Figure 5.5). We will meet some of these receptors again later in the chapter as they are the target for antihypertensive drugs.

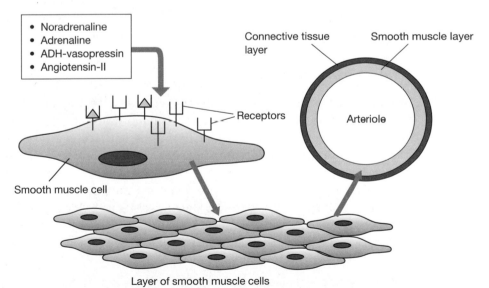

Figure 5.5 Control of arterioles by neurotransmitters and messengers such as noradrenaline, adrenaline, angiotensin-II and ADH-vasopressin, each binding to its own specific receptors resulting in vasoconstriction.

Cardiac output (heart rate × stroke volume)

Cardiac output, the amount of blood ejected from the left ventricle in one minute, is determined by two factors – heart rate and stroke volume. If either heart rate or stroke volume increase, then cardiac output will increase (and so BP increases). If either heart rate or stroke volume decrease, then cardiac output will decrease (and so BP decreases). Heart rate is the rate that the heart beats each minute, so the faster the heart beats, the more blood it will pump. Stroke volume is the amount of blood ejected from the left ventricle with each beat (around 70 ml at rest). A more forceful contraction, such as occurs during exercise, will eject even more blood – up to 100 ml or so in a normal individual. Sympathetic stimulation increases both heart rate and stroke volume – as does an increase in circulating adrenaline from the adrenal gland.

DID YOU KNOW . . . that during a marathon race, the average runner's heart will have beaten 35,000 times? Typical heart rate will be around 150 beats per minute and the heart will pump 100 ml of blood with each beat. This means that if a runner takes four hours to finish, their heart will have pumped over 3500 litres of blood! At rest, 1200 litres of blood would be typical in four hours.

Another factor in the control of stroke volume is the amount of blood that is returning to the heart. This is known as the **preload**. For example, during exercise when the heart is working harder, more blood returns to the heart. This increase in end-diastolic volume or preload causes the heart muscle to stretch more, resulting in a more forceful contraction and a larger stroke volume. This effect is called **Starling's law** after Ernest Starling, an English physiologist who worked at University College London in the early part of the last century.

The baroreceptor reflex

Arterial blood pressure is monitored by pressure sensors in the circulatory system called **baroreceptors**, the most important of which are found on the **aortic arch** and the **carotid sinus** (a dilation of the internal **carotid artery** that supplies the brain). These stretch receptors monitor changes in blood pressure and send nervous signals to the **cardiovascular control centre** in the **medulla**, a region of the brain stem. The medulla regulates blood pressure by adjustments to the cardiac output of the heart and the peripheral resistance of the systemic arterioles. This process is called the baroreceptor reflex. We will now examine the response of the baroreceptor reflex to decreases and increases in blood pressure.

Baroreceptors are small regions on the aorta and carotid sinus that respond to changes in the stretch of the vessel walls as blood pressure fluctuates by sending signals to the cardiovascular control centre in the brain stem.

A decrease in blood pressure can have many causes such as haemorrhage, dehydration, heart attack and even just standing up too quickly. This drop in BP is detected by the baroreceptors which send signals to the cardiovascular control centre in the medulla via **afferent** neurons. The medulla then increases sympathetic activity in the circulatory system. This has the effect of increasing both the stroke volume and heart rate which increases the cardiac output. Sympathetic activity also causes vasoconstriction in the peripheral arterioles which increases systemic vascular resistance (Figure 5.6). All of these contribute to an increase in blood pressure.

If you remember our formula for blood pressure, $BP = CO \times SVR$, where cardiac output is defined by $CO = HR \times SV$, you can see that the baroreceptor response increases all of the factors involved in blood pressure regulation. Heart rate, stroke volume and systemic vascular resistance all increase and consequently, so does blood pressure.

Afferent neurons are those that travel from the periphery into the central nervous system (CNS). Neurons that travel out of the CNS into the periphery are called **efferents**. A way of memorising these two words is that **E**fferents **E**xit the CNS.

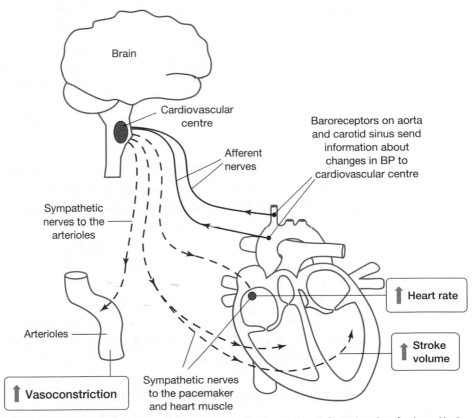

Figure 5.6 Control of blood pressure via the baroreceptor reflex showing factors that respond to a fall in blood pressure.

ANOTHER WAY TO PICTURE THIS

Remember we compared the arterial system to a long, thin balloon with a small hole in the end. If pressure in the balloon fell you would blow harder and more regularly (increase cardiac output) and pinch the other end to reduce the amount of air escaping (increase systemic vascular resistance).

So how does the body respond to an *increase* in blood pressure which is normally an indication of exercise? Obviously, a response that reduced cardiac output would be undesirable as it would limit our ability to exercise. However, complex mechanisms in the central nervous system suppress the baroreceptor response and selective vasodilation occurs that redistributes blood to the exercising muscles. This lowers systemic vascular resistance so that blood pressure only increases moderately, even though cardiac output may have doubled.

CASE STUDY

After major thoracic surgery, Graham appears to be recovering satisfactorily when you notice that his pulse rate has increased, he looks pale and feels cold to the touch. You check his blood pressure and this is normal. What might be causing the observed changes?

Comment on case study An unexplained increase in a patient's heart rate needs investigating. It may be that Graham is anxious but it could be that his blood pressure is falling and he is compensating by increasing his heart rate. If he looks pale and has cold skin, this could be a sign of vasoconstriction of the peripheral arterioles in the skin. The fact that his BP is normal may be because his compensatory mechanisms are currently sufficient to maintain his blood pressure. There could be several problems that are causing his blood pressure to fall, but after major surgery, internal bleeding is a possibility.

A QUICK RECAP on the short-term regulation of blood pressure

- The short-term regulation of blood pressure is largely determined by two factors – cardiac output (CO) and systemic vascular resistance (SVR).
- Cardiac output in turn is determined by heart rate and stroke volume.
- If blood pressure falls then the body will increase CO and SVR.
- The baroreceptor reflex responds to a fall in blood pressure by activating the sympathetic nervous system. This acts on the heart and systemic arterioles, increasing both CO and SVR and so blood pressure is increased.
- Various chemical messengers such as adrenaline, angiotensin-II and ADH-vasopressin can bind to receptors on the arterioles and cause vasoconstriction, so increasing SVR.

The long-term regulation of blood pressure

The baroreceptor response is primarily there to respond to short-term changes in blood pressure. Long-term regulation involves adjusting sodium (Na^+) levels

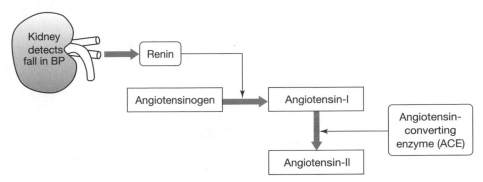

Figure 5.7 How angiotensin-II is produced in response to a fall in blood pressure.

in the blood and this is done by the kidneys via the **renin–angiotensin** (RA) **system**.

The kidneys respond to any fall in blood pressure or a reduction in the flow of blood by releasing the enzyme **renin** into the blood. This enzyme converts a circulating protein called **angiotensinogen** into **angiotensin-I**, which is further modified by **angiotensin-converting enzyme** (ACE) into **angiotensin-II** (Figure 5.7).

Angiotensin-II is the key protein in the long-term regulation of blood pressure. It circulates in the blood and has several actions, all of which act together to increase blood pressure.

1 Angiotensin-II causes the adrenal glands to release the hormone **aldosterone**. This hormone acts on the kidneys causing them to conserve sodium (Na^+) in the body by reducing the amount of Na^+ lost in the urine. The conservation of Na^+ by the kidneys increases levels of Na^+ in the blood and this increases the amount of water that the blood will hold. As the blood volume increases, the amount of blood returning to the left ventricle increases and so does the preload. With more blood in the left ventricle, the heart's muscle fibres become more stretched and under Starling's law, the force of contraction increases. The stroke volume increases and this in turn increases cardiac output and blood pressure. This might be more clearly explained in a flow chart (Figure 5.8).

Yes (before you ask) the renin–angiotensin system is complicated but ACE inhibitors, one of the most common group of drugs used in the treatment of high blood pressure, heart failure, etc., act on the RA system. You need to understand this system in order to understand the action of ACE inhibitors.

2 Angiotensin-II is a potent vasoconstrictor that binds to angiotensin-II receptors on the smooth muscle cells of blood vessels and causes them to constrict. Vasoconstriction increases systemic vascular resistance and as we know from our blood pressure formula, when SVR increases, so does blood pressure.

3 Angiotensin-II promotes the release of the hormone **ADH-vasopressin** from the anterior pituitary gland in the brain. ADH stands for **antidiuretic hormone**

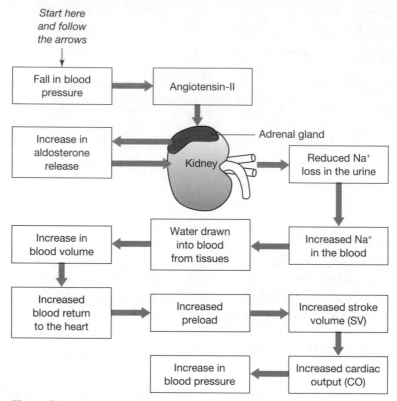

Figure 5.8 How angiotensin-II (released in response to a fall in blood pressure) acts on the kidneys to increase blood volume and blood pressure.

and as the name implies, causes the kidneys to conserve water by reducing the amount of urine produced. Conserving water in the body helps to maintain blood volume and also blood pressure. The **vasopressin** part of the name gives a clue to the hormone's other action; it acts on smooth muscle of the blood vessels as a vasoconstrictor and so increases systemic vascular resistance – and blood pressure.

Well, that's about all you need to know about blood pressure in order to understand how the various antihypertensive drugs work. However, before this we will need to understand something about the cause of hypertension and its consequences.

Do I really need to know all this stuff about blood pressure regulation?

Yes, you definitely need to understand the mechanisms of blood pressure regulation. Most antihypertensive drugs interfere with these mechanisms, decreasing either cardiac output or systemic vascular resistance. If you don't understand the principles of regulation then you will not understand how antihypertensive drugs work.

A QUICK RECAP on the long-term regulation of blood pressure

- The long-term regulation of blood pressure is primarily by the renin–angiotensin system.

- When blood pressure falls, renin is released by the kidneys and this converts angiotensinogen into angiotensin-I which is finally converted into angiotensin-II by an angiotensin-converting enzyme.

- Angiotensin-II causes the hormone aldosterone to be released, and this makes the kidneys conserve sodium which increases blood volume, cardiac output, and therefore blood pressure.

- Angiotensin-II causes vasoconstriction of the arterioles resulting in an increase in systemic vascular resistance, and therefore blood pressure.

- Angiotensin-II promotes the release of the hormone **ADH-vasopressin** that causes the kidneys to reduce urine production and so conserve body fluids, helping to maintain blood pressure. ADH-vasopressin also increases SVR.

5.2 The pathology of hypertension

This will be a rather short section because over 90 per cent of cases of hypertension are of unknown origin. If you look in most books you will see most cases of hypertension described as **idiopathic** which simply means that the cause is unknown. Idiopathic hypertension is also known as primary or **essential hypertension**. Hypertension is defined as having a systolic pressure of over 140 mmHg and a diastolic pressure over 90 mmHg. The problem gets more serious as pressures increase. Mild hypertension, between 140 and 159 mmHg may initially be treated by changes in lifestyle, but more aggressive pharmacological treatment is needed as the problem gets worse.

> **KEY FACT**
>
> The cause of most **hypertension** is unknown. This means that we are more often treating the symptom than the cause.

Pathologies that cause an increase in cardiac output, or an increase in systemic vascular resistance such as neurological or hormonal imbalances are the ones most likely to increase blood pressure – but in most cases the cause is unknown. Environment and lifestyle factors such as stress, smoking and obesity can exacerbate hypertension. Drugs such as alcohol, non-steroidal anti-inflammatory drugs (NSAIDS), steroids and even liquorice can also result in an increase in blood pressure. Particular ethnic groups may be more prone to hypertension, for example people of Afro-Caribbean origin are more likely to be hypertensive than other races. Age is an important risk factor as people are more likely to suffer from hypertension as they get older, especially after the age of 55 when around two-thirds of the population are hypertensive.

IN PRACTICE

An interesting cause of hypertension in some individuals is a phenomenon known as '**white coat syndrome**' where their blood pressure increases rapidly when a nurse or doctor takes their blood pressure. As soon as the procedure stops, their blood pressure returns to normal!

Secondary hypertension is generally due to problems such as kidney disease, but the cause is seldom identifiable.

People who are hypertensive may initially experience few symptoms, but over many years prolonged high blood pressure can damage organs, especially the brain, kidneys and cardiovascular system, and may result in **haemorrhagic stroke**, renal failure and myocardial infarction (heart attack). The development of atherosclerosis is accelerated in people with high blood pressure, especially if they are also diabetic. The heart itself can be affected over time as it is put under strain having to pump against high aortic pressure. The heart muscle gradually thickens and dilates, sometimes resulting in heart failure.

Because hypertension is generally symptomless, many people are not aware that they have high blood pressure until a routine check-up by their GP reveals the problem.

Haemorrhagic stroke is when the blood supply to the brain is interrupted by a bleed in the brain itself, often caused by the rupture of a blood vessel. Other types of stroke include **ischaemic stroke** that is caused by the formation of a blood clot in the arteries of the brain.

CASE STUDY

Jane is 75 and has been diagnosed as hypertensive. When her GP checks Jane's blood pressure it is around 160/90 mmHg and he tells her that she may need to start taking drugs to reduce it. Strangely, when Betty the community nurse visits Jane at home and checks her BP, it is much lower – why might this be?

Comment on case study Jane's blood pressure may actually be within acceptable limits most of the time but the stress of visiting her GP's surgery may increase it to the point where she appears hypertensive – so-called 'white coat syndrome'. Betty, the community nurse, is visiting Jane in the relaxed surroundings of her own home and so is able to take her BP without stress temporarily increasing the reading.

5.3   Drugs used in the treatment of hypertension

The treatment of hypertension can be quite difficult because the choice of treatment for an individual patient is determined by so many factors, including the severity of the problem, the underlying pathology, other problems such as diabetes, the age and even the ethnic origins of the individual – not to mention their response to previous medication.

For mild hypertension where there are no complications, changes in lifestyle rather than drug therapy are to be preferred. Giving up smoking, losing weight, eating plenty of fruit and vegetables, taking exercise, and cutting down on both salt and excessive alcohol consumption can reduce blood pressure sufficiently to remove the necessity of long-term antihypertensive therapy. However, where blood pressure is significantly elevated or where there are complications such as diabetes, antihypertensive drugs may be the only solution.

Many drugs are used to treat hypertension and the choice of which is best for a particular patient is a clinical decision that must be made by the prescriber in accordance with local and national guidelines. In the UK, the **National Institute for Health and Clinical Excellence** (NICE) provide guidance on the treatment and care of people with hypertension and other diseases and conditions within the National Health Service. Currently, ACE inhibitors (or angiotensin receptor blockers if ACE inhibitors are not tolerated) are the drugs of choice, followed by calcium channel blockers then thiazide-type diuretics. Patients over 55 years of age or of Afro-Caribbean descent (any age) are not recommended ACE inhibitors as initial treatment for reasons discussed shortly.

CASE STUDY

Mark is a reasonably fit and healthy, non-smoking 45 year old but at a recent visit to his GP, his blood pressure was found to be 150/90 mmHg. This was confirmed after home monitoring and Mark returned to his GP for a discussion as to the best course of treatment. What would you suggest?

Comment on case study If Mark is reasonably fit and healthy then he is probably asymptomatic with regard to his high blood pressure. It is good that he does not smoke as this would tend to increase his BP. Initially, lifestyle changes should be tried before resorting to drugs. Salt intake should be reduced, fresh fruit and vegetable intake increased and Mark should be encouraged to exercise more. Swimming, jogging or cycling might be suitable activities.

Principles for the treatment of hypertension

If you remember back a few pages, you will recall that there was a simple formula that explained the factors regulating blood pressure:

$$BP = CO \times SVR$$
(Blood pressure = Cardiac output × Systemic vascular resistance)

Table 5.2 Showing effect of main antihypertensive drugs on the factors that determine blood pressure

Drug group	Action on SVR and CO	
	SVR	CO
ACE inhibitors and related drugs	Reduction	Reduction
Angiotensin-II receptor blockers	Reduction	Reduction
Thiazide diuretics	None	Reduction
Calcium channel blockers*	Reduction	Reduction
Beta-blockers	None	Reduction
Alpha-blockers	Reduction	None

* Action varies with type of calcium channel blocker.

where cardiac output is defined by

$$CO = HR \times SV$$

(Cardiac output = Heart rate × Stroke volume)

Remember that the body's response to a fall in blood pressure is to increase cardiac output and systemic vascular resistance which returns the blood pressure to its normal level. We are now going to use this formula again to explain the action of antihypertensive drugs but instead of aiming to increase blood pressure we are going to reduce it.

> **KEY FACT**
>
> **Antihypertensive drugs** work by a variety of mechanisms but eventually all reduce either cardiac output or systemic vascular resistance – or both.

Table 5.2 shows the action of the main antihypertensive drugs on factors that determine blood pressure. Note that the reduction in either factor, systemic vascular resistance or cardiac output, will reduce blood pressure.

Drug groups in the treatment of hypertension

Antihypertensive group 1: angiotensin-converting enzyme (ACE) inhibitors (and related drugs)

These drugs are used to treat essential hypertension and some are also used for heart failure. This group of drugs includes *captopril, cilazapril, enalapril, fosinopril, imidapril, lisinopril, moexipril, perindopril, quinapril, ramipril* and *trandolapril*. *Aliskirin* is a related drug, introduced relatively recently, that has a slightly different action to the other ACE inhibitors.

ACE inhibitors interfere with the renin–angiotensin system that regulates long-term blood pressure. Remember that the body responds to a fall in blood pressure by converting angiotensin-I into angiotensin-II via angiotensin-converting enzyme (ACE). Angiotensin-II circulates in the blood where it has various actions that together increase blood pressure.

1 Aldosterone production is increased and this increases blood sodium, blood volume and so blood pressure.

2 Angiotensin-II also acts as a general vasoconstrictor and so increases systemic vascular resistance.

3 Angiotensin-II stimulates the release of ADH-vasopressin and, as well as acting as a vasoconstrictor, this hormone conserves water by reducing urine output.

ACE inhibitors are similar in molecular structure to angiotensin I and so bind to the active site of angiotensin converting enzyme and thus block its activity, preventing the conversion of angiotensin-I to angiotensin-II. Circulating levels of angiotensin-II fall and so does blood pressure (Figure 5.9).

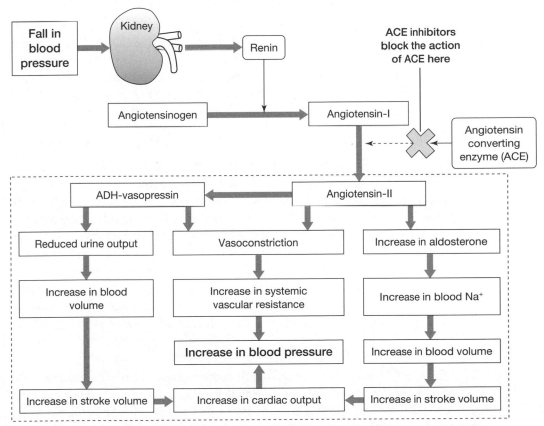

Figure 5.9 ACE inhibitors block the production of angiotensin-II, inhibiting the processes contained within the dotted line, and so reducing blood pressure.

> **IN PRACTICE**
>
> Remember that the NICE guidelines do not recommend the use of ACE inhibitors for patients over 55 years or of Afro-Caribbean descent of any age. The reason for this is that renin production by the kidney reduces with age and is naturally very low in Afro-Caribbean people so ACE inhibitors are less effective because the renin–angiotensin system will play a lesser part in overall blood pressure regulation.

Side-effects Persistent dry cough is a common side-effect. ACE inhibitors not only inhibit angiotensin-converting enzyme but other enzymes in the lungs resulting in an accumulation of **bradykinin** in the bronchioles. Bradykinin irritates the tissues, resulting in a dry cough. ACE inhibitors can also cause hypotension, especially in patients on diuretics. Any drug strong enough to counteract the action of the body's powerful compensatory mechanisms is likely to tip the balance in the other direction and cause an excessive fall in blood pressure.

Antihypertensive group 2: renin inhibitors

Aliskirin is currently in a group on its own. A relatively recent drug, it interferes with the renin-angiotensin system but not by inhibiting the action of angiotensin converting enzyme. Instead it blocks the action of renin itself so preventing it from converting angiotensinogen into angiotensin-I. The reduction in circulating levels of angiotensin-I results in a corresponding reduction in angiotensin-II and from here the effect is the same as that of an ACE inhibitor.

Antihypertensive group 3: angiotensin-II receptor blockers (ARBs)

These drugs are used to treat essential hypertension and some are also used for heart failure. This group includes *candesartan, eprosartan, irbesartan, losartan, olmesartan, telmisartan* and *valsartan*. Patients who find the cough produced by many ACE inhibitors unacceptable, may be better able to tolerate these drugs.

Angiotensin-II is a potent vasoconstrictor that causes an increase in systemic vascular resistance. Angiotensin-II targets angiotensin-II receptors on the smooth muscle cells that surround the arteries and arterioles. This causes the muscle cells to contract resulting in vasoconstriction of the peripheral arterioles and an increase in SVR. Angiotensin-II receptor blockers bind to and block the Angiotensin-II receptor and therefore reduce the vasoconstrictive effect of angiotensin-II (Figure 5.10).

Antihypertensive group 4: thiazide diuretics

There are several groups of drugs that produce diuresis, including **loop diuretics**, **thiazide diuretics** and **potassium sparing diuretics**. Of these the thiazide diuretics are considered one of the first drugs of choice for hypertension. The group includes *bendroflumethiazide, chlortalidone, cyclopenthiazide, indapamide, metolazone* and *xipamide*.

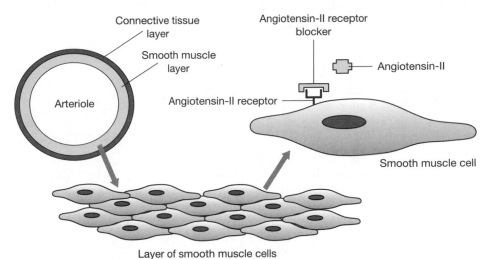

Figure 5.10 Angiotensin-II receptor blockers (ARBs) block angiotensin-II receptors from the vasoconstrictive action of angiotensin-II.

Diuretics stimulate the production of urine. In the kidneys, the blood is filtered in small filtration units called **nephrons** and, after processing, the filtered fluid becomes urine. This means that as urine production increases so more fluid is removed from the blood and therefore blood volume decreases. This in turn reduces preload in the left ventricle and a lower preload means a lower stroke volume and a lower cardiac output. Diuretics work by a common mechanism, altering the osmotic balance in the kidney and so increasing the amount of urine produced. The mechanism whereby the kidneys control the body's water balance is very complex. Instead, we will outline the basic principles of diuresis and leave you to get a more detailed explanation of how the kidneys work from any general physiology book.

> **KEY FACT**
>
> **Diuretics** increase urine production and this reduces blood volume. As blood volume drops, so does cardiac output and blood pressure.

The kidneys are primarily a collection of millions of tiny tubes called nephrons. Within each nephron is a filtration unit called a **glomerulus**, a group of capillaries supplied with blood from a renal arteriole. The pressure in the glomerulus forces fluid from the blood through the glomerulus wall into the **Bowman's capsule** (Figure 5.11). This fluid is called **filtrate** and contains body waste such as urea and other small soluble molecules in the blood but not blood cells or plasma proteins. Around 140 litres of filtrate is produced each day by the millions of nephrons, but most of the water content of the filtrate is reabsorbed back into

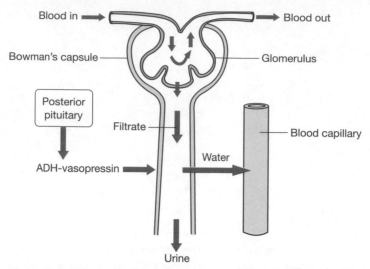

Figure 5.11 Schematic diagram of a kidney nephron. Water is reabsorbed from the filtrate under the influence of the pituitary hormone ADH-vasopressin.

the blood. This leaves between 1 and 2 litres of urine to pass from the nephrons, down the **ureters** and into the **urinary bladder** from where it is voided from the body as urine.

The amount of filtrate produced each day is fairly constant but the amount of urine varies, depending on the hydration state of the individual. You have no doubt noticed that when you have been exercising on a hot day you do not produce much urine. On the other hand, if you have been out visiting friends and drinking tea or coffee socially, then you might be quite desperate to get home (and relieved when you do so). Urine production is controlled by the hormone ADH-vasopressin released by the posterior pituitary gland and its production increases as the body becomes more dehydrated. ADH-vasopressin is released into the bloodstream and acts on the **tubules** of the **nephron**, causing them to become more permeable to water, which leaves the nephron and is picked up by adjacent capillaries. The more ADH is produced, the more water is reabsorbed from the filtrate and the less urine is produced (Figure 5.11).

DID YOU KNOW . . . that the common dandelion *Taraxacum officinalis* has been used for centuries as a diuretic? The fresh leaves also taste nice in salads but there is a tradition that it causes nocturnal enuresis, hence the French name for dandelion, *pissenlit* – literally translated as urinating in bed!

Diuretics inhibit water reabsorption from the filtrate, so more is lost as urine. They do this by blocking sodium and chloride ion pumps on the wall of the nephron. This has the effect of upsetting the osmotic balance in the tissue surrounding the nephron and this decreases the rate at which water is reabsorbed. As less water is absorbed from the filtrate, more water is lost as urine, and this causes a reduction in blood volume and blood pressure – as described above.

Side-effects As with most other antihypertensives, thiazide diuretics can tip the balance the other way, resulting in hypotension. **Hypokalaemia** (low potassium) and **hyponatraemia** (low sodium) can also be a problem as a consequence of interfering with the ionic balance of the kidney. See the current BNF for a full list of side-effects.

IN PRACTICE

Hypokalaemia and hyponatraemia can result from the use of diuretics or from severe sweating, vomiting or diarrhoea. Hypokalaemia can sometimes cause abnormal heart rhythms. Symptoms of hyponatraemia (low sodium) can include nausea, headaches and confusion.

CASE STUDY

Jim is 65 and was diagnosed with high blood pressure 5 years ago. He had gone to see his GP because of a persistent dry cough (despite having no chest infection) and was also concerned about his kidneys because he needed to go to the toilet 'for a wee' two or three times during the night. His current medication is *ramipril* – 5 mg once daily and, more recently, *bendroflumethiazide* – 5 mg once daily. Jim usually takes his medication around 9 o'clock at night with his evening cocoa.

Comment on case study It could be the ACE inhibitor that is causing the problem dry cough. Jim might be able to switch to another antihypertensive drug such as an angiotensin-II receptor blocker. In fact it was unusual for Jim to have been prescribed an ACE inhibitor as patients over 55 are less likely to respond to an ACE inhibitor (NICE guidelines). It is probably the thiazide diuretic that is causing Jim to visit the toilet during the night, which is why these diuretics are usually taken first thing in the morning to avoid this problem.

Antihypertensive group 5: calcium channel blockers

Calcium channel blockers (CCBs) are a diverse group of drugs and exert their effects by different mechanisms. Drugs in this group that are licensed for the treatment of hypertension include *amlodipine, diltiazem, felodipine, isradipine, lacidipine, lercanidipine, nicardipine, nifedipine, nisoldipine* and *verapamil*.

How come there are so many different types of drugs in this group?

If any group of drugs is successful this creates a market and manufacturers will develop their own drug to exploit that market. Also, as soon as a popular drug goes out of copyright then rival manufacturers will start to produce their own version. Currently, nine different drug manufacturers are producing *diltiazem*.

Calcium channel blockers act on calcium ion channels in various cells that have an important role in determining blood pressure. These cells include the **myocytes** (muscle cells of the heart), the heart's **pacemaker cells** and the smooth muscle cells of the arterioles. Calcium channels play an important role in the operation of these structures and blocking the channels with CCBs results in a fall in blood pressure – but by a variety of mechanisms. Ultimately, they reduce cardiac output or systemic vascular resistance and so reduce blood pressure.

The heart's muscle cells The entry of calcium ions into the myocytes of the heart initiates their contraction. CCBs block Ca^{2+} channels in the myocytes' cell membrane and this reduces the cells' ability to contract. A reduction in the force of contraction reduces stroke volume.

The heart's pacemaker cells The entry of Ca^{2+} ions into the heart's pacemaker cells is also an important determinant of heart rate, so blocking the Ca^{2+} channels results in a slowing of the heart. A reduction in heart rate reduces cardiac output.

The arterioles The contraction of smooth muscle cells surrounding arterioles involves the entry of ions through Ca^{2+} channels in the cell membrane. As CCBs block the Ca^{2+} channels, contraction is inhibited and vasodilation promoted (Figure 5.12). Vasodilation reduces systemic vascular resistance.

Blocking calcium channels in the cardiovascular system therefore results in a reduction in systemic vascular resistance, heart rate and stroke volume and all of these factors combine to reduce blood pressure. There are small differences in the chemical structure of the various CCBs that result in differences in their action. For example, *nifedipine* acts mainly on the smooth muscle of the arterioles, causing them to dilate while *verapamil* reduces cardiac output and *diltiazem* is intermediate in its actions.

Side-effects There are many, including constipation which is most likely caused by CCBs blocking Ca^{2+} channels in the smooth muscle that encircles the gut. This reduces its contractility and therefore motility, leading to the sluggish passage of

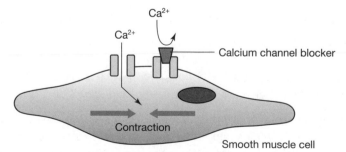

Figure 5.12 The entry of calcium into the smooth muscle cells surrounding the arterioles induces contraction, so blocking Ca^{2+} channels with CCBs induces relaxation and vasodilation.

food through the gastro-intestinal system. See the current BNF for a full list of side-effects.

REALITY CHECK

Can you explain three ways that blocking calcium channels in the arterioles and heart can reduce blood pressure?

Antihypertensive group 6: beta-blockers

Examples of this group include *acebutolol, atenolol, bisoprolol, carvedilol, metoprolol* and *propranolol*. Selected members of this group of drugs are also used for angina and arrhythmias and as an adjunct in heart failure. For general antihypertensive therapy, current NICE Guidelines relegate β-blockers to the drug of fourth choice behind thiazide diuretics, calcium channel blockers and ACE inhibitors.

We examined the anti-anginal action of beta-blockers in Chapter 4 and saw that they block β_1 receptors on the heart, thus reducing its responsiveness to activity by the sympathetic nervous system. As this keeps the heart rate low and reduces the workload of the heart, it is very useful in patients with angina and heart failure. However, the action of beta-blockers in hypertension is not straightforward because sympathetic activity is minimal during rest, so blocking the receptors to sympathetic activity has little effect on the resting heart. The exact mechanism is not fully understood but it is now believed that beta-blockers primarily exert their antihypertensive action by inhibiting the release of renin from the kidneys. We have already examined the renin–angiotensin system in some detail when we looked at ACE inhibitors, so it should be evident why a reduction in renin produces a fall in blood pressure.

Unwanted effects β_2 adrenergic receptors in the bronchioles are targets for adrenaline agonists such as *salbutamol*. Beta-blockers are essentially β_1 antagonists targeting the heart, but they can also block the β_2 receptors in the lungs, isolating these receptors from the therapeutic action of *salbutamol*. This is why beta-blockers are contra-indicated for asthma patients.

Antihypertensive group 7: alpha-adrenoceptor blockers

These drugs are generally used in combination with other hypertensives rather than on their own as mono-therapy. Selected members of the group are also indicated for **benign prostatic hyperplasia** (enlarged prostate gland) and congestive heart failure. The group includes *doxazosin, indoramin, prazosin* and *terazosin*.

The arterioles respond to a variety of vasoconstrictive chemical substances released in the body including, as we have seen, angiotensin-II, ADH-vasopressin and adrenaline. Both circulating adrenaline and noradrenaline, released as a neurotransmitter by the sympathetic nervous system, bind to alpha-1 (α_1) receptors on the arterioles with the same effect. Blocking these receptors antagonistically means that neither adrenaline nor noradrenaline can bind and this results in relaxation of the smooth muscles of the arterioles and vasodilation (Figure 5.13).

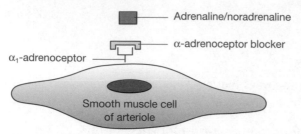

Figure 5.13 Alpha-adrenoceptor blockers such as **doxazosin** isolate smooth muscle cells of the arterioles from the vasoconstrictive action of adrenaline and noradrenaline.

These drugs also have a relaxing effect on the smooth muscle of the bladder and prostate gland, explaining their usefulness in the treatment of benign prostatic hyperplasia.

A QUICK RECAP on drugs used in the treatment of hypertension

- ACE inhibitors such as **captopril** block the action of angiotensin converting enzyme that converts angiotensin-I to angiotensin-II.

- Angiotensin-II causes vasoconstriction and an increase in cardiac output (by increasing blood volume) – so blocking the production of angiotensin-II – resulting in vasodilation and a fall in cardiac output. Together this causes a fall in BP.

- **Aliskirin**, a renin inhibitor, produces the same effect as ACE inhibitors by blocking the enzyme renin.

- Angiotensin-II binds to receptors on smooth muscle cells in the arterioles and causes vasoconstriction. Angiotensin-II receptor blockers such as **candesartan** prevent angiotensin-II binding to its receptors and this results in vasodilation, a decrease in SVR and a fall in BP.

- Thiazide diuretics such as **bendroflumethiazide** increase the production of urine and thus reduce the blood volume, which reduces cardiac output and thus BP.

- Calcium channel blockers such as **amlodipine** have effects on the smooth muscle cells in the arterioles and the heart. Both systemic vascular resistance and cardiac output are reduced along with BP.

- Beta-blockers such as **atenolol** have a poorly understood action as antihypertensives, but probably inhibit the release of renin which reduces the activity of the renin–angiotensin system and thus BP.

- Alpha-adrenoceptor blockers such as **doxazosin** block α_1-adrenergic receptors on the smooth muscle cells in the arterioles from the vasoconstrictive effect of adrenaline and noradrenaline. This results in vasodilation, a decrease in SVR and a fall in BP.

RUNNING WORDS

Here are some of the technical terms that were included in this chapter.
Read through them one by one and tick them off when you are sure that you
understand them.

ADH-vasopressin p. 121

Afferent p. 118

Aldosterone p. 121

Angiotensin-converting
enzyme (ACE) p. 121

Angiotensin-I p. 121

Angiotensin-II p. 121

Angiotensinogen p. 121

Antidiuretic hormone
p. 121

Aortic arch p. 118

Baroreceptors p. 118

Benign prostatic
hyperplasia p. 133

Bowman's capsule p. 129

Bradykinin p. 128

Cardiac output (CO)
p. 114

Cardiovascular control
centre p. 118

Carotid artery p. 118

Carotid sinus p. 118

Diastolic p. 112

Diuretics p. 129

Efferents p. 119

Essential hypertension
p. 123

Filtrate p. 129

Glomerulus p. 129

Haemorrhagic stroke
p. 124

Heart rate p. 114

Hypertension p. 110

Hypokalaemia p. 131

Hyponatraemia p. 131

Idiopathic p. 123

Ischaemic stroke p. 124

Loop diuretics p. 128

Medulla p. 118

Myocytes p. 132

Nephron p. 129

Pacemaker cells p. 132

Potassium sparing
diuretics p. 128

Preload p. 118

Pulsatile p. 112

Radial Artery p. 112

Radius p. 112

Renin p. 121

Renin-angiotensin (RA)
system p. 121

Secondary hypertension
p. 124

Sphygmomanometer
p. 112

Starling's law p. 118

Stroke volume p. 114

Systemic vascular
resistance (SVR)
p. 114

Systolic p. 112

Thiazide diuretics p. 128

Thoracic cavity p. 112

Tubules p. 130

Ureters p. 130

Urinary bladder p. 130

Vasopressin p. 122

'White coat syndrome'
p. 124

REFERENCES AND FURTHER RECOMMENDED READING

All recommended websites are open access (but free registration is sometimes required).

National Centre for Health and Clinical Excellence (Guidelines for the treatment of hypertension) – http://www.nice.org.uk/Guidance/CG34

Opie, L.H. and Gersh, B.J. (2008) *Drugs for the Heart* (7th edition). Saunders.

Student, B.M.J. – http://student.bmj.com/topics/clinical/cardiovascular_medicine.php

British Heart Foundation – http://www.bhf.org.uk/

Bandolier: hypertension – http://www.medicine.ox.ac.uk/bandolier/

Your turn to try

That was quite a testing chapter to work through but hypertension is a very common problem and you will find patients on antihypertensive medication in many clinical scenarios. Not only is it important to understand the pharmacology of hypertension but the chapter will also have given you a good refresher in the physiology of blood pressure regulation. Let's see how much you have remembered and understood of Chapter 5.

Try answering these questions, first from memory, then check the answers on page 285.

1 When you are checking someone's pulse in (say) the radial artery, is the pulse rate the same as heart rate?

2 Pressure in the arteries fluctuates between systole and diastole – which of these two is the higher pressure?

3 If cardiac output falls, what happens to blood pressure?

4 Name three substances carried in the blood that result in vasoconstriction.

5 What is the neurotransmitter released by sympathetic neurons that causes vasoconstriction?

6 If blood pressure falls because of haemorrhage, what would you expect to happen to heart rate?

7 If there is a general vasodilation of the systemic arterioles, what happens to blood pressure?

8 Name three effects of angiotensin-II.

9 ACE inhibitors inhibit the production of angiotensin-II and by so doing reduce aldosterone production – why might this reduce blood pressure?

10 Do diuretics increase or decrease the amount of water reabsorption in the tubules of the nephron?

11 Are diuretics most likely to lead to hypernatraemia or hyponatraemia?

12 What is the effect of blocking calcium channels in arteriole smooth muscle cells?

13 By what mechanism might CCBs cause constipation?

14 How do beta-blockers reduce blood pressure?

15 Why are beta-blockers contra-indicated in asthma?

Answers to questions on page 111

1 Aorta.
2 Right.
3 Atria.
4 Systole.
5 Oxygenated.
6 Vein.

Chapter 6

Inflammation and the management of pain

AIMS

By the time you have finished the chapter you will understand . . .

1 The **physiology** – the anatomy and physiology of pain pathways
2 The **pathology** – inflammation and how it may result in pain
3 The **pharmacology** – action of the major drug groups used to attenuate inflammatory and trauma-induced pain

CONTENTS

The chapter contains some brief case studies and finishes off with some self-test questions in order that you can make sure that you have understood the physiology, pathology and pharmacology of pain and pain relief.

IN PRACTICE

You will encounter patients who are experiencing pain and being treated for it. In surgical wards, patients will have undergone operations that may be causing post-operative pain. In medical wards, patients may have infections and conditions such as cancer that cause pain. Midwives will be looking after women experiencing the pain of childbirth. In the community, elderly patients may be experiencing pain from chronic problems such as arthritis or sciatica. Pain is often the reason that patients seek medical help, so one of the first stages in the diagnosis of a problem is to ask the patient to describe the source and type of pain. This is why you need to understand the nature of pain and also the drugs that are used to help people who are in pain.

Introduction

Undoubtedly, everyone reading this chapter will have had some experience of pain. Hopefully the pain will have been fairly minor, arising from the bumps, grazes, toothache and nettle stings that most of us experience at one time or another. For others the pain may have been more severe, caused by accidents such as falling off a bicycle or perhaps the pain associated with childbirth. Most people would agree that pain is unpleasant and it is fortunate that medical science has developed techniques in pain management that reduce it to bearable levels. This has in itself led to major advances in surgical techniques that would be impossible without adequate pain control. Less than 200 years ago, operations were conducted without anaesthetic (or with copious amounts of alcohol), patients were forcefully restrained and surgeons had to operate very quickly indeed. Contrast that with the complex, life-saving procedures that modern surgeons perform, thanks to advanced anaesthesia.

Many philosophers have pondered on the subject of pain, asking why we should have to experience such a seemingly unnecessary and unpleasant phenomenon. Pain appears to serve no function except to aggravate an already unpleasant situation such as an injury or infection, so why should pain pathways have evolved in humans and probably all animals that possess a nervous system?

The answer becomes apparent when we consider the fate of those few individuals who are born without the ability to experience pain, a condition called **congenital analgesia**. You might think that it would be wonderful never to have toothache again or experience wasp or nettle stings but there is a downside. If you do not know that you are about to sustain an injury then you may not take the appropriate action to avoid that injury. Think what happens when you accidentally touch a hot domestic iron or a hotplate on a kitchen cooker. Almost before your skin touches the hot object you experience an unpleasant sensation and quickly withdraw your hand. Imagine what would happen if you did not experience that pain – there could have been quite a lot of tissue damage before you discover that your hand was on fire! Similarly, if your finger touches a thorn on a rose bush, you feel the pain as the thorn pricks your finger and very quickly move your finger away. If you did not experience that sharp immediate pain then the thorn could easily pierce your flesh which could possibly become infected. Pain also teaches us to avoid potentially painful and thus dangerous situations such as fierce dogs, swarms of bees and chain saws.

Pain is also a useful mechanism for informing us that we have sustained an injury or developed an infection. We can then take the appropriate action to protect the injury from further damage, clean and dress the wound and possibly seek medical assistance.

In this chapter we will explore the way that the body detects pain and relays that information to the brain where the pain is conceptualised. Inflammation is associated with many clinical situations such as injury, infection and surgical procedures so we explore the nature of inflammation and how it may result in pain. Finally, we look at a very important but diverse group of drugs that relieve or prevent pain. These drugs range from over-the-counter analgesics for minor to moderate pain such as **paracetamol** to opioids such as **morphine** that are used to control severe pain. Because inflammation is a common source of pain we examine the mechanism of action of the non-steroidal anti-inflammatory drugs (NSAIDs) such as **ibuprofen** and also anti-inflammatory corticosteroids such as **prednisolone**. Finally, we examine the local anaesthetics such as **lidocaine**, which is widely used in dentistry and minor surgery.

WHERE ARE WE STARTING FROM?

In this chapter we will be discussing the nervous system and how it transmits pain signals to the brain. We will also be examining the action of drugs on pain pathways so it is important that you understand the basic layout of the nervous system and how nervous impulses are transmitted along neurons (nerve cells).

Let's start off with a short quiz to find out how much you know before we begin:

1 The nervous system can primarily be divided into two divisions, the central nervous system and the . . . ?

_____

2 Do afferent neurons carry information into or out of the central nervous system?

_____

3 What is the difference between a neuron and a nerve?

_____

4 Name the two divisions of the autonomic nervous system.

_____

5 Motor neurons control which type of tissues?

_____

Answers are at the end of the chapter on page 161.

How did you do? If you got all five correct then fine – you obviously have a basic knowledge of the nervous system. Otherwise, you might do well to open your favourite physiology book and brush up on the nervous system to make sure you understand the first section of this chapter. This is not the easiest of the body's systems to learn but you will need a good grasp of it to understand how the drugs work.

6.1 The physiology of pain and pain pathways

The experience of pain differs between individuals and will vary according to the nature of the noxious stimulus, previous exposure and the reaction to pain of that individual. The definition of pain accepted by most clinical practitioners goes something like:

> 'Pain is whatever the patient informs you that they are experiencing.'

This is because no one can truly appreciate the pain that another person is experiencing. Some people are (or say they are) relatively impervious to pain while others seem to react excessively to any painful stimulus – no matter how small. This means that whatever your belief about a patient's pain, he or she is the only one who really knows what it is like, so you have to respect the patient's description of the experience.

We generally divide pain into two types – **nociceptive** and **neuropathic** – and each type requires different clinical approaches and drugs.

Nociceptive pain usually has an identifiably physiological cause such as inflammation or injury. The pain from this source is transmitted along pain neurons into the spinal cord and up to the brain where the pain is conceptualised. Drugs that block the transmission of nervous impulses along the pain pathways will prevent pain messages from reaching the brain. This is perhaps the most common cause of pain and its treatment is perhaps the most straightforward.

Neuropathic pain is caused by neurological dysfunction that results in the perception of pain. Various conditions can affect nerves and these can cause neuropathic pain as a consequence of the problem. These conditions include **trigeminal neuralgia**, **shingles**, **multiple sclerosis** and **diabetic neuropathy**. Neuropathic pain can manifest itself in **hyperalgesia**, which is the experience of severe pain from a stimulus that would normally cause only slight discomfort. **Paresthesia** is another manifestation – unpleasant or painful feelings such as pins and needles with no apparent stimulus – and **allodynia** is pain from a stimulus that should not normally cause pain. Symptoms such as depression and anxiety may also result from neuropathic pain. The physiology, pathology and treatment of neuropathic pain is often uncertain and problematical so we will concentrate in Chapter 6 on nociceptive pain and give a brief résumé of the drugs that are used to treat neuropathic pain at the end of the chapter.

> **KEY FACT**
>
> **Nociceptive pain** generally has an identifiable cause such as injury and involves pain signals travelling to the brain along pain pathways. Neuropathic pain is caused by problems within the nervous system itself and it is often more difficult to identify the cause of this type of pain.

Acute and chronic pain

Another way that pain can be categorised is by separating it into **acute** or **chronic**. These divisions refer to the length of time that the pain is experienced by the individual and makes no reference to its intensity. Acute pain is short term and lasts a definite period of time before, for example, an injury is resolved and the pain subsides. Chronic pain is defined as pain that lasts more than six months. It may be neuropathic or nociceptive in origin, and caused perhaps by a long-term degenerative disease such as osteoarthritis.

> **DID YOU KNOW . . .** that the word 'chronic' is widely misused as meaning severe when it simply refers to the long duration of a problem or pain? The word comes from the Ancient Greek word *khronos* meaning time. This is the origin of words such as *chronometer* (accurate clock) and *chronological* (in date order).

The neuroanatomy of pain

Nociceptive pain is transmitted along a relay of neurons, from the site of injury, into the spinal cord and up to the brain where the signals are conceptualised as pain. At the **distal** end of afferent **nociceptive neurons** (pain neurons) there are **nociceptors** (pain receptors) that respond to painful stimuli such as heat, mechanical pressure and chemical stimulation. Once stimulated, these neurons send nervous impulses into the spinal cord and from there to the brain (Figure 6.1).

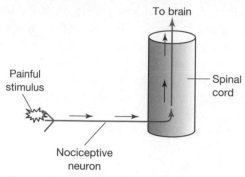

Figure 6.1 A noxious stimulus is transmitted along an afferent nociceptive neuron into the spinal cord and from there to the brain.

Distal refers to the point on an anatomical structure furthest away from the centre of the body. If you think of the human arm, the fingers are distal to the elbow. A point nearer to the centre is **proximal**, so the elbow is proximal to the fingers.

Nociceptors, found in most tissues, are nerve endings that respond to chemical, thermal and mechanical stimuli. There are various types of nociceptors and various types of nociceptive neurons, some of which transmit fast impulses representing sharp, well-localised pain while others, perhaps associated with inflammation, transmit slower impulses that signify a more diffuse, dull aching type of pain.

Let us now follow in some detail the neural pathways that take pain signals from the site of injury into the spinal cord and up to the brain. Firstly, we have the painful stimulation, perhaps a minor cut to a finger. The nociceptor is stimulated by the tissue damage and this initiates nervous impulses that are sent along the arm via the afferent nociceptive neuron and then into the spinal cord. Arriving via the **dorsal root** of the spinal cord, the nociceptive neuron sends signals across a **synapse** (nerve junction) to an ascending neuron that ascends to the **thalamus** in the brain where the signal crosses another synapse and finally reaches the **cerebral cortex** via a **thalamic-cortical** neuron (Figure 6.2). Some of the neurons that convey dull, aching pain ascend to the brain by a slightly different route but, essentially, all pain pathways lead eventually to the cerebral cortex where the information is processed into a form of conscious pain experience.

Synapse - where two neurons meet you will find a synapse. Nervous impulses jump from one neuron to another across these interesting structures by means of chemical messengers called neurotransmitters.

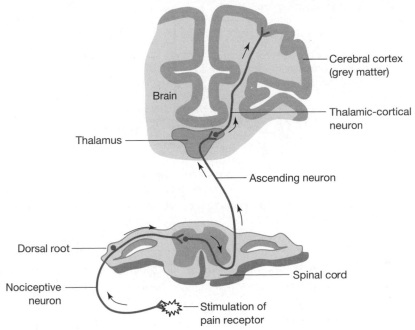

Figure 6.2 Nociceptive pathways conveying pain signals from a site of injury to the cerebral cortex of the brain.

REALITY CHECK

Are you sure that you understand how pain is transmitted to the brain along pain pathways? Imagine that you prick your finger on a thorn – can you trace the pathway for pain information along your own arm, into your spinal cord and up to your brain? Although it appears to be your finger that hurts, do you understand that it is your brain interpreting the pain signals?

The body's own analgesic system

The body has evolved its own analgesic system that becomes activated when an animal is injured. This in-built analgesia provides short-term relief from pain that enables an animal to escape from predators or extract themselves from a dangerous situation without being crippled with pain. The mechanism is not fully understood but it is believed to originate deep within the brain from where efferent neurons descend down the brain stem and spinal cord where they meet with incoming afferent nociceptive neurons. Here the descending neurons release **opioid-like peptides** which block the transmission between the afferent nociceptive neurons and so inhibit the experience of pain (Figure 6.3). As we will see later in the chapter, this in-built analgesic system is utilised by opioid drugs such as *morphine* and *codeine* so it is important that we spend a few moments to explain how the opioid-like peptides work on the synapses in the spinal cord.

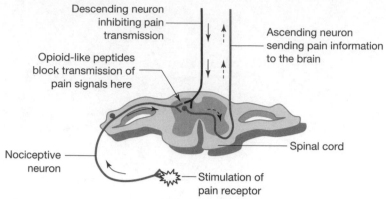

Figure 6.3 Descending neurons inhibit pain transmission pathways in the body's own analgesic system.

DID YOU KNOW . . . that opioid-like substances are released during sustained strenuous exercise such as running or cycling? It is believed that these substances cause a sense of well-being or even euphoria that some endurance athletes experience and may even lead to them becoming addicted to exercise.

The synapse

Let us briefly examine how synapses operate because they are key targets for opioid drugs. When a nervous impulse arrives at the axon terminal of a neuron, it cannot simply jump to the next neuron because at the junction between the neurons there is a small gap that forms part of a structure called the synapse (Figure 6.4). The synapse comprises the axon terminal of the transmitting neuron

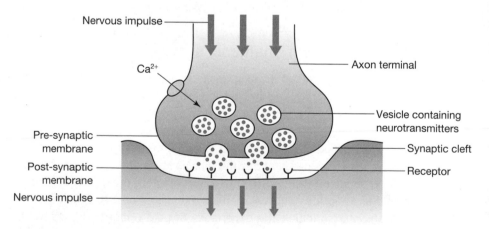

Figure 6.4 Schematic diagram of a synapse. Nervous impulses are transmitted across the synapse via neurotransmitters (note that some types of neurotransmitter inhibit the forward transmission of nervous impulses).

and the cell membrane of the receiving neuron, separated from each other by a small gap called the **synaptic cleft**. Communication across the synaptic cleft is via neurotransmitters released by the transmitting neuron. As you can see from Figure 6.4, the neurotransmitters are prepacked into small bubble-like structures called **vesicles**. When a nervous impulse arrives at the end of the transmitting neuron, this causes calcium ions to enter the terminal which stimulates the release of the neurotransmitters. These diffuse across the cleft and bind to receptors on the **post-synaptic membrane** of the cell receiving the message and this either stimulates or inhibits the receiving cell.

These synapses are complicated. Are they targeted by any other drugs beside opioids?

Synapses are indeed complex, perhaps one of the most complex structures in the body. They are targeted by many drugs, especially those used to treat mental health problems. Our four protein drug targets – receptors, ion channels, enzymes and carrier proteins are all found in synapses and can be targeted by various drugs.

A QUICK RECAP on the physiology of pain and pain pathways

- We can divide pain into various categories: nociceptive and neuropathic describe the origin of the pain; chronic and acute describe the duration of the pain.
- In nociceptive pain, signals are transmitted along a relay of nociceptive neurons from the origin of the injury or disease, up the spinal cord to the brain.
- The body has its own analgesic system that reduces pain immediately after injury.
- The analgesic system inhibits pain transmission in the synapses of the spinal cord.

6.2 The pathology of inflammation

When you hit your thumb with a hammer or cut yourself with the kitchen knife, you notice the area surrounding the injury becomes red, warm, swollen and painful – this is inflammation. You might think that what you are observing is the random consequence of tissue damage but this is not the case. Inflammation is a carefully programmed, non-specific immune response to injury, noxious chemical agents and microbial pathogens. The inflammatory response occurs immediately after trauma or infection and prevents the spread of pathogens, minimises further damage to cells and tissue and finally enhances repair and healing.

Inflammation manifests itself by the following symptoms:

- Redness
- Heat
- Swelling
- Pain
- Alteration of function

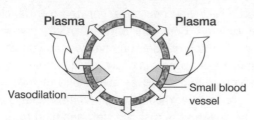

Figure 6.5 Small blood vessels in the inflamed area dilate and become leaky. This increases blood flow to the area making it red and warm. Plasma leaking into tissues causes swelling.

The inflammatory response involves three key processes:

1 The vasodilation of small blood vessels in the area of damage, resulting in an increase in blood flow.

2 An increase in **vascular permeability** that causes **plasma** (the liquid, non-cellular part of the blood) to leak from small blood vessels into the area of damage.

3 The emigration of **neutrophils** (white blood cells) from the blood into the damaged area.

These processes can explain some of the symptoms of inflammation mentioned earlier. For example, vasodilation increases the blood flow to the damaged area and blood makes the area red and warm (Figure 6.5). Inflammation results in plasma leaking from the small blood vessels into the area of damage or infection and this causes **oedema** (swelling). This can also cause pressure on pain neurons and results in the dull, aching pain familiar in inflammation. Swelling can also impede muscle and joint movement and cause loss of function. Chemicals released in inflammation can add to the sensation of pain, and these will be discussed later.

> **Vascular permeability** – Vascular relates to the blood vessels and permeability is a measure of how easily fluid will pass through a membrane, etc. In this case an increase in vascular permeability means that the blood vessels become leaky.

The leaking of plasma from the small blood vessels brings **plasma proteins** into intimate contact with the damaged area. These proteins include the **clotting proteins** that help to stop bleeding and various immune proteins that help to destroy any microbes that may have been introduced into the area with the injury. Also introduced are proteins called **kinins** that promote vasodilation, increase the permeability of blood vessels and stimulate pain receptors. We will meet the kinins later when we examine how inflammation causes pain.

CASE STUDY

Geoff was playing football when he tripped and twisted his ankle. Still in his football strip, he presents in casualty with an ankle that is severely swollen, red and warm to the touch. It is also extremely painful and Geoff can't bear to put his foot on the ground. What are the processes triggered by the sprain that have caused Geoff's symptoms?

Comment on case study This is a classic presentation of inflammation. The tissue damage caused by the accident has triggered the inflammatory process resulting in oedema, loss of function and pain. Vasodilation has brought extra warm blood to the area giving it a flushed, red appearance. The extent of the damage needs proper clinical assessment but often sprains look and feel worse than they actually are. Hopefully, with rest, anti-inflammatories and TLC, Geoff will be back playing football in a few weeks' time.

Mast cells

Mast cells are key components in the inflammatory response. They are found in connective tissue adjacent to blood vessels and injury or stimulation by the immune system causes mast cells to release various mediators (locally acting chemicals) – Figure 6.6. Mast cells are part of the **granulocyte** family of white blood cells, so-called because they contain granules of prepacked mediators that can be released very quickly once the mast cell is stimulated to do so, perhaps by injury.

Mast cells release various mediators by degranulation, including **histamine**. Histamine causes vasodilation and also increases the permeability of small blood vessels, making the area red, warm and swollen – as discussed above. Other

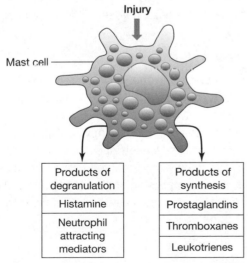

Figure 6.6 Mast cells release mediators either by degranulation or more gradually by synthesis.

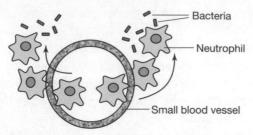

Figure 6.7 Neutrophils are attracted by mediators released by mast cells and migrate from the blood to the area of inflammation where they phagocytose bacteria.

mediators released by mast cells attract circulating **neutrophils** from the blood which squeeze through the walls of the small blood vessels and migrate towards the area of inflammation. Here, the neutrophils mature and **phagocytose** micro-organisms that may have caused the infection or have been introduced into a wound during the initial injury (Figure 6.7).

> **Phagocytose** – literally translated means eating cells. Neutrophils and macrophages are large immune cells that engulf and destroy bacteria.

Other chemical mediators have to be synthesised and consequently are released some time after histamine, and these include **prostaglandins, thromboxanes** and **leukotrienes**. These mediators are very important pharmacologically because there are many groups of drugs that are targeted at either blocking their production or inhibiting their action.

REALITY CHECK

Can you explain how inflammatory processes result in the key symptoms of inflammation, namely swelling, heat, redness, pain and loss of function?

Prostaglandins

Prostaglandins are important mediators in the inflammatory process. They are members of a large family derived from **arachidonic acid** (a fatty acid) and are found in most tissues of the body. Prostaglandin biochemistry is complex, as are the actions of prostaglandins themselves. They belong to a family that includes prostaglandins, thromboxanes and leukotrienes that have important roles, unconnected with inflammation in maintaining cell and tissue homoeostasis.

Prostaglandin E_2 (PGE_2) is the main prostaglandin involved in inflammation. It is secreted by mast cells and other immune cells, and reinforces the action of histamine and bradykinin, resulting in

- Vasodilation of small blood vessels
- Increased vascular permeability
- Stimulation of nociceptive neurons.

PGE$_2$ also plays a less-well-defined role in the transmission of pain signals in the spinal cord and in the **hypothalamus** of the brain. It can affect the body's thermostat, resulting in **pyresis** (fever). Prostaglandins also have many roles unconnected with inflammation, including the maintenance of the **gastric mucosa** (lining of the stomach), the inhibition of gastric acid secretion and sleep regulation.

> **Hypothalamus** - situated at the base of the brain, the hypothalamus has a key role in maintaining the internal environment of the body. The hypothalamus regulates the sympathetic and parasympathetic nervous system as well as the release of pituitary hormones.

Because anti-inflammatory drugs inhibit prostaglandin synthesis, it is necessary to examine briefly how they are produced by mast and other immune cells. The raw material is the phospholipid membrane of the cell. This is converted into **arachidonic acid**, then into a **cyclic endoperoxide** and finally into a prostaglandin or thromboxane (Figure 6.8).

The key enzyme in this process is a cyclo-oxygenase (COX) that has arachidonic acid as its substrate. There are several forms of cyclo-oxygenase but the two that have known pharmacological significance are COX-1 and COX-2. Prostaglandins and thromboxanes are produced extensively in the body and have many roles unconnected with inflammation. These are produced by the enzyme COX-1 which can be thought of as a housekeeping enzyme producing prostaglandins and thromboxanes that are involved in many important body functions such as ion transport, gastric acid regulation, synaptic regulation, blood clotting, etc. COX-2 is produced in large amounts during inflammation and itself produces large amounts of prostaglandins in the inflamed area, in particular PGE$_2$.

> **KEY FACT**
>
> COX-1 is an enzyme that is produced in many tissues where it produces prostaglandins and thromboxanes involved in homeostasis. COX-2 is an enzyme found primarily in inflamed tissues where it produces prostaglandin E$_2$ that contributes to the symptoms of inflammation.

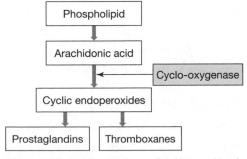

Figure 6.8 Outline pathway for the synthesis of prostaglandins and thromboxanes.

Leukotrienes are closely related to prostaglandins and thromboxanes and have been implicated in asthma. Their synthesis uses a similar pathway but does not involve the cyclo-oxygenase enzyme. Their role in inflammation is still being determined but they are known to activate and sensitise some white blood cells and cause bronchoconstriction.

Yes, prostaglandin chemistry is quite complex but it is the major target of non-steroidal anti-inflammatory drugs (NSAIDs) such as *diclofenac* and *ibuprofen*. Thromboxanes are targets of *aspirin* in the prevention of clotting and the action of leukotrienes is inhibited by anti-asthma drugs such as *montelukast* and *zafirlukast*.

The role of prostaglandins in inflammatory pain

There are two key mechanisms whereby prostaglandin E_2 increases pain. Firstly, PGE_2, along with histamine and bradykinin, increases vascular permeability and the resulting swelling increases pressure in the inflamed area that stimulates nociceptive neurons (Figure 6.9).

Prostaglandin E_2 also increases pain by making nociceptive neurons more sensitive to the bradykinin produced in inflammation (Figure 6.10). Bradykinin is a potent stimulator of nociceptive neurons and its action is enhanced by the presence of PGE_2.

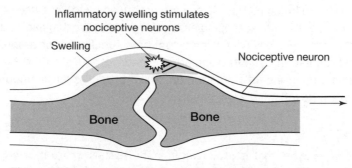

Figure 6.9 Pressure from inflammatory swelling stimulates nociceptive neurons.

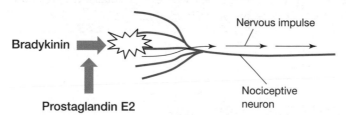

Figure 6.10 PGE_2 sensitises nociceptors to the action of bradykinin.

A QUICK RECAP on the pathology of inflammation

● Inflammation is a programmed response to infection or injury.

● The key signs of inflammation are redness, heat, swelling, pain and alteration of function.

- Vasodilation brings more blood to the inflamed area making it red and warm.

- Plasma leaks out of small blood vessels into tissues making them swollen and painful, and reducing their ability to function.

- Mast cells and other immune cells produce histamine and prostaglandins that are key players contributing to vasodilation and causing small blood vessels to leak plasma.

- Prostaglandin E_2 is the main inflammatory prostaglandin, produced in a pathway where COX-2 is a key enzyme.

- The body produces many prostaglandins in other tissues that are unconnected with inflammation, produced in a pathway where COX-1 is the key enzyme.

6.3 Drugs used in the management of inflammation and pain

Non-steroidal anti-inflammatory drugs (NSAIDs)

There are many non-steroidal anti-inflammatory drugs (NSAIDs) available including *aspirin*, *ibuprofen*, *naproxen*, *flurbiprofen*, *diclofenac* and *indometacin*. All NSAIDs have a similar action, reducing inflammation, swelling and pain by inhibiting the production of prostaglandins, especially PGE_2. The key target for NSAIDs is the cyclo-oxygenase enzyme COX-2 – the form that is produced during inflammation and contributes to the production of copious amounts of PGE_2. This prostaglandin contributes to the increase in vascular permeability that allows plasma to leak from the blood into the area of inflammation. The resulting swelling can increase pressure on nociceptive neurons, stimulating them and causing the familiar inflammatory aching pain. PGE_2 also sensitises nociceptors to the pain-producing mediator bradykinin, contributing to the pain experienced. For these reasons, it is obviously desirable to block the action of COX-2 and so reduce the production of PGE_2 to help relieve inflammatory pain.

> **KEY FACT**
>
> Non-steroidal anti-inflammatory drugs block the enzyme COX-2, found primarily in inflamed tissues where it is part of the pathway that produces prostaglandin E_2.

Side-effects The side-effects of NSAIDs are numerous and vary between patients in severity and frequency. The gastro-intestinal tract (GIT) appears to be particularly vulnerable, resulting in discomfort, diarrhoea, nausea and sometimes ulceration

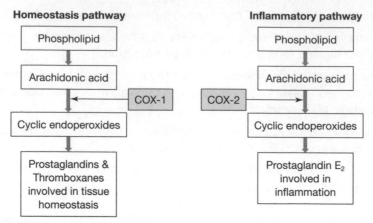

Figure 6.11 Showing how closely related are the inflammatory and non-inflammatory pathways that produce prostaglandins. Drugs targeted at COX-2 may also bind to and inhibit the action of COX-1.

and bleeding. Some patients exhibit hypersensitivity to NSAIDs and can experience rashes and oedema. NSAIDs can worsen their symptoms for some asthmatics.

Prostaglandins have a role in regulating stomach acid and also in the maintenance of the gastric mucosa, so the inhibition of prostaglandins by NSAIDs explains their adverse gastro-intestinal effects. Figure 6.11 shows how closely related are the pathways that produce inflammatory and non-inflammatory prostaglandins. The two forms of cyclo-oxygenase, COX-1 and COX-2, are very similar in structure so it is little wonder that NSAIDs targeted at the inflammatory enzyme COX-2 may also block and inhibit the action of the non-inflammatory enzyme COX-1 that maintains tissue homoeostasis.

IN PRACTICE

You have a patient who has been prescribed *ibuprofen* after minor surgery. Can you explain to the patient, in easy-to-understand terms, how the drug works and what side-effects to look out for?

IN PRACTICE

Although some NSAIDs are available OTC (over-the-counter) from chemists and even supermarkets, they are not as safe as many would believe. This is especially so in elderly patients who are more susceptible to bleeding as a side-effect of NSAIDs and for whom the consequences of bleeding are more likely to be serious. NSAIDs also increase risk in elderly patients suffering from cardiac or renal disease.

Selective COX-2 inhibitors

This group of drugs includes *celecoxib* and *etoricoxib* and has the same basic mechanism of action as other NSAIDs such as *ibuprofen* and *diclofenac*. The key difference is that this group has a high specificity for COX-2 and so is useful in the treatment of chronic inflammatory diseases such as osteoarthritis and rheumatoid arthritis where the long-term use of conventional NSAIDs proves problematical. Because these drugs are highly specific for COX-2, they do not inhibit COX-1 appreciably and therefore should not affect the production of those non-inflammatory prostaglandins involved in normal tissue homeostasis. In particular, they should not cause gastro-intestinal problems as can the long-term use of conventional NSAIDs.

Unfortunately these drugs have had a chequered history and over the past few years several have been withdrawn because of concerns over their safety due to evidence that they caused an increase in the rate of heart attacks and liver toxicity. At the time of writing (2009) only *celecoxib* and *etoricoxib* remain on licence and neither of these drugs is recommended for patients with coronary artery disease.

Paracetamol

Paracetamol is a non-anti-inflammatory, non-steroidal that has mainly **antipyretic** (fever reducing) and analgesic properties. Its mechanism of action is by no means well understood but it is suggested that it inhibits a variant of a cyclo-oxygenase enzyme in the central nervous system. Because it has little effect on normal pro-staglandin production it is relatively free of those side-effects commonly caused by conventional NSAIDs, in particular gastro-intestinal irritation.

Although the short-term use of *paracetamol* at therapeutic doses produces relatively few side-effects, liver damage can unfortunately occur at only two to three times the therapeutic dose.

CASE STUDY

Anne is 60, has been admitted to hospital for hip replacement and complains of post-operative pain. You are aware that she suffers from angina and has had a stomach ulcer and are worried that conventional NSAIDs such as *diclofenac* are likely to cause gastric bleeding. Would a COX-2 inhibitor such as *etoricoxib* be suitable to help ease Anne's pain?

Comment on case study The use of conventional NSAIDs such as *diclofenac* where someone is at risk from gastro-intestinal bleeding is not advised and even selective COX-2 inhibitors should only be used with caution. However, Anne also has angina, which is indicative of coronary artery disease. This means that she is at risk of a heart attack so COX-2 inhibitors are definitely not suitable for her as they increase the risk of coronary problems. *Paracetamol*, which is not associated with gastric bleeding or a heart attack, might be a better choice.

IN PRACTICE

Would you feel able to discuss with colleagues the different actions and side effects of analgesics such as NSAIDs, selective COX-2 inhibitors and paracetamol?

Anti-inflammatory steroids

Anti-inflammatory steroids mimic the action of natural **glucocorticoids** such as **hydrocortisone** and **corticosterone** – stress hormones secreted by the adrenal gland in response to injury, stress, severe infection and pain. They have a general immuno-suppressive activity, as well as increasing the metabolism of carbohydrate and protein and reducing inflammation. They increase the supply of glucose, triglycerides and amino acids to ensure the nutrient supply to key organs such as the brain and to provide materials for the repair of tissues. Although it may seem strange, glucocorticoids also limit the inflammatory response during injury, presumably to limit damage that may occur from excessive activity in the immune system.

Anti-inflammatory corticosteroids include *beclometasone*, *betamethasone*, *cortisone*, *hydrocortisone*, *prednisolone* and *dexamethasone* that have a variety of uses including the reduction of inflammatory pain in rheumatoid arthritis, the prevention of asthma attacks, the treatment of psoriasis and also immuno-suppression after transplantation to prevent rejection.

Being derivatives of cholesterol, corticosteroids are lipid in nature and can therefore pass through the cell membrane without requiring a transporter protein. They act deep inside the cell, in the nucleus where they bind to receptors that control the production of proteins. Their anti-inflammatory action is thought to be due to the fact that they reduce the release of **cytokines**, which are chemical signals released by immune cells such as neutrophils, mast cells and macrophages. As we saw earlier in the chapter, inflammation results in pain, so any group of drugs that have an anti-inflammatory action will reduce nociceptive pain.

IN PRACTICE

The long-term use of systemic glucocorticoid drugs can suppress the activity of the adrenal gland resulting in reduced levels of natural glucocorticoids. If steroid drugs are withdrawn abruptly, this can leave the adrenal cortex insufficient time to recover, and circulating glucocorticoids, both synthetic and natural, can be so low as to cause severe hypotension and even death. Patients on long-term systemic steroids should carry a Steroid Treatment Card that explains this risk.

The long-term use of systemic glucocorticoids is problematical. Elevated blood glucose levels can result in type-2 diabetes, and immunosuppression can result in infections. Bone metabolism can be adversely affected, resulting in **osteoporosis**, thinning of the bones, and growth can be retarded in children. Metered dose inhalers used in asthma deliver corticosteroids in a formulation that produces the maximum anti-inflammatory effect in the bronchioles with the minimum systemic effect, thus allowing their safe long-term use.

> **Osteoporosis** is a condition where the bones become porous and weak. It is more common in women and often progresses more quickly after the menopause when female hormone levels begin to decline.

Opioid analgesics

Morphine and its relatives make up the opioid analgesics, perhaps the strongest and most effective pain killers in current use. It is closely related to heroin, an illegal narcotic, but as *morphine* is less lipid soluble, it is slower to cross the blood–brain barrier and produce the euphoric effects of heroin. *Morphine* is obtained from opium, the sap of the poppy *Papaver somniferum* that is grown in a band of south Asian countries from Afghanistan to Thailand. Current opioids include *morphine*, *buprenorphine*, *codeine*, *diamorphine*, *fentanyl*, *methadone*, *pethidine* and *tramadol*. Each opioid drug has its own benefit with regard to speed of onset, duration of effect and side-effects, but *morphine* itself is generally thought of as the most valuable analgesic for severe pain.

> **DO YOU KNOW...** the difference between an *opioid* and an *opiate*? The two terms are often used interchangeably but there is a technical difference. *Opiates* are the natural alkaloids derived from opium whereas the term *opioid* refers to all drugs with a morphine-like action, including semi-synthetics such as *fentanyl*.

As we saw earlier in this chapter, the body possesses its own analgesic system which damps down incapacitating pain immediately after injury. This involves the release of opioid-like peptides which block the transmission of nervous impulses between the afferent nociceptive neurons, thus inhibiting the experience of pain. Efferent neurons from the brain descend the spinal cord to synapse with the afferent nociceptive neurons in the dorsal horn. Here they release the opioid-like peptides such as **β-endorphin**, **dynorphin** and **enkephalins** that block the synaptic transmission of the afferent neurons and thus reduce the experience of pain.

The opioid-like peptides inhibit synaptic transmission by binding to opioid receptors on the pre-synaptic membrane and the post-synaptic membrane of the synapse. On the pre-synaptic membrane they inhibit the opening of the calcium channels and so prevent the release of the neurotransmitter that sends the signal to the receiving neuron. On the post-synaptic membrane, the opioid-like

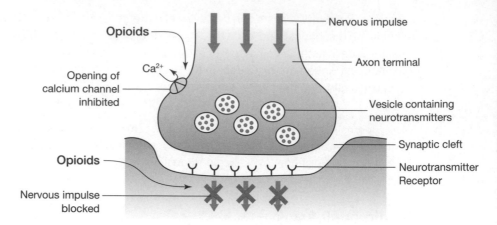

Figure 6.12 Opioids bind to opioid receptors (not shown) and inhibit the transmission of nervous impulses across the synapses between pain neurons.

peptides bind to opiate receptors and make the membrane less responsive to stimulation by neurotransmitters. As *morphine* and other opioid drugs are similar in molecular structure to the opioid-like peptides, they bind to the same opioid receptors and produce the same effect – inhibition of the pain transmission across the synapse (Figure 6.12).

Opioids: side-effects

Any drug that has such a strong effect on the nervous system will almost inevitably be associated with unwanted effects. There appear to be opioid receptors in various parts of the body and it is the action of opioid drugs on these receptors that is responsible for most of the side-effects. Nausea and vomiting, especially after initial administration, can be a problem, as can respiratory depression with some opioids, believed to be due to a reduction in the sensitivity of respiratory centres in the brain stem to carbon dioxide, the main driver of breathing. A decrease in gastro-intestinal motility is another problem with opioids, especially *codeine*.

> ### CASE STUDY
>
> Stan has terminal cancer and is receiving palliative care at home, which includes oral *morphine* to help with the pain. He is relatively pain free with the prescribed medication but complains of constant nausea and also constipation. What would you advise?

Comment on case study Nausea and constipation are common side-effects of *morphine* but Stan's pain is under control, which is important for patients with terminal cancer. Pain control in palliative care is a specialist area and any changes to his medication should be done with caution. Exercise might help with the constipation but this might not be practical in the circumstances, so dietary changes or a laxative might help. There are anti-nausea drugs such as *metoclopramide* and *haloperidol* that might help with the nausea.

REALITY CHECK

Can you explain the action of the opioid-like peptides and how they help to reduce the experience of pain? Can you explain how opioid drugs mimic the action of opioid-like peptides and produce the same effect?

Local anaesthetics

All local anaesthetics in current use are derivatives or analogues of cocaine, a drug extracted from leaves of the coca plant, *Erythroxylum coca,* grown in South America. For thousands of years South American Indians have chewed the leaves of the coca plants to relieve fatigue in the harsh climate of the high Andes. Its numbing effect was later utilised in Europe to relieve pain in surgical procedures. Current local anaesthetics in common use include **lidocaine**, **bupivacaine**, **levobupivacaine, prilocaine, ropivacaine** and **tetracaine**.

Local anaesthetics are relatively uncomplicated in their action, blocking nervous impulses in the nociceptive neurons. All nervous impulses depend on sodium channels opening in the neuron membrane. As the nervous impulse arrives at a section of the neuron membrane, sodium channels open and this allows the impulse to move to the next section of membrane where sodium channels open, allowing the nervous impulse to move to the next section of membrane . . . and so on (Figure 6.13). Potassium channels are also involved in the nervous impulse, but we will concentrate on the sodium channels as they are the main targets for local anaesthetics.

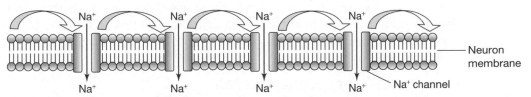

Figure 6.13 A nervous impulse travels along a neuron as Na^+ channels open in the cell membrane.

Local anaesthetics block Na^+ channels in the membranes of nociceptive neurons. This prevents the nervous impulse travelling along the nociceptive neuron and the subsequent neurons in the pain pathway on its way to the brain. If pain signals do not reach the brain, the individual will not experience any pain (Figure 6.14).

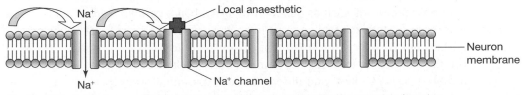

Figure 6.14 A local anaesthetic blocks Na^+ channels and halts the nervous impulse.

Local anaesthetics block conduction primarily in the small-diameter afferent nociceptive neurons rather than the larger motor neurons, and this means that motor control is less affected than pain perception. However, some loss of motor function occurs, depending on procedure and dose, as anyone who has tried to eat or talk after a local anaesthetic for dental work will testify.

Epidurals are useful for a variety of procedures where anaesthesia of a large region of the body is required or where general anaesthesia is contra-indicated or undesirable, for example in childbirth. Epidurals can be used in general surgical procedures in the pelvic region or legs, for example hip replacement. *Lidocaine* and *bupivacaine* are used at concentrations that produce dense sensory block and usually induce moderate to dense motor block. For analgesia during labour, *bupivacaine* is used at lower concentrations than for surgical procedures and is popular as it produces less interference with motor function.

IN PRACTICE

Epidurals are very effective for operations where a general anaesthetic is undesirable. The epidural is delivered by injection into the epidural space surrounding the spinal cord. Needless to say, this is a procedure requiring special training and is invariably performed by an anaesthetist.

The most significant unwanted effects result from local anaesthetics entering the circulatory system, and to prevent this problem they are often combined with adrenaline – a vasoconstrictor which inhibits blood flow to the area being anaesthetised – thus limiting seepage of the drug into the general circulation.

Drugs used for neuropathic pain

Neuropathic pain is pain caused by neurological dysfunction rather than the stimulation of nociceptive neurons by injury, inflammation, etc. This makes pain relief problematical because the pain is not following the normal neural pain pathways that can be targeted by conventional analgesics. Sometimes analgesics such as *paracetamol*, non-steroidal anti-inflammatory drugs (NSAIDs), *codeine*, etc., have an effect on neuropathic pain but the results are unpredictable. Anti-depressants such as the tricyclic, *amitriptyline*, can be effective but they work by a poorly understood mechanism, separate to their action on depression. Anti-epileptic drugs such as *gabapentin*, *pregabalin*, *carbamazepine* and *sodium valproate* inhibit excitable neurons in epilepsy and have a similar action in neuro-pathic pain. Generally the treatment of neuropathic pain can be difficult because the mechanism that causes the pain is poorly understood. It is, therefore, often a matter of carefully trying different drugs and monitoring their effects to see which works best.

A QUICK RECAP on drugs used in the management of inflammation and pain

- Non-steroidal anti-inflammatory drugs (NSAIDs) target the COX-2 enzyme responsible for producing the inflammatory prostaglandin PGE_2.

- NSAIDs can also inhibit COX-1 enzyme that has a variety of non-inflammatory functions in the body. This may produce some of the side-effects associated with NSAIDs.

- *Paracetamol* is a widely used analgesic drug without an anti-inflammatory action.

- Anti-inflammatory steroids such as *prednisolone* act by suppressing activity in the immune cells involved in inflammation.

- Opioid drugs mimic natural opioid-like peptides that work in the synapses between nociceptive neurons to dampen pain after injury.

- Local anaesthetics block sodium ion channels in nociceptive neurons, and this inhibits the transmission of pain signals to the brain.

RUNNING WORDS

Here are some of the technical terms that were included in this chapter. Read through them one by one and tick them off when you are sure that you understand them.

Acute p. 141	Epidurals p. 158	Paresthesia p. 141
Allodynia p. 141	Gastric mucosa p. 149	Phagocytose p. 148
Antipyretics p. 153	Glucocorticoids p. 154	Plasma p. 146
Arachidonic acid p. 148	Granulocyte p. 147	Plasma proteins p. 146
β-endorphin p. 155	Histamine p. 147	Post-synaptic
Cerebral cortex p. 142	Hydrocortisone p. 154	membrane p. 145
Chronic p. 141	Hyperalgesia p. 140	Prostaglandins p. 148
Clotting proteins p. 146	Hypothalamus p. 149	Proximal p. 141
Congenital analgesia	Kinins p. 146	Pyresis p. 149
p. 138	Leukotrienes p. 148	Shingles p. 140
Corticosterone p. 154	Multiple sclerosis p. 140	Synapse p. 142
Cyclic endoperoxide	Neuropathic pain p. 140	Synaptic cleft p. 145
p. 149	Neutrophils p. 146	Thalamic-cortical p. 142
Cytokines p. 154	Nociceptive neurons	Thalamus p. 142
Diabetic neuropathy	p. 141	Thromboxanes p. 148
p. 140	Nociceptive pain p. 140	Trigeminal neuralgia
Distal p. 141	Nociceptors p. 141	p. 140
Dorsal root p. 142	Oedema p. 146	Vascular permeability
Dynorphin p. 155	Opioid-like peptides p. 143	p. 146
Enkephalins p. 155	Osteoporosis p. 155	Vesicles p. 145

REFERENCES AND FURTHER RECOMMENDED READING

All recommended websites are open access (but free registration is sometimes required).

The Oxford Pain Internet Site (access from) – http://www.medicine.ox.ac.uk/bandolier/

The British Pain Society – http://www.britishpainsociety.org/

Your turn to try

Now you have finished reading this chapter it is time to find out how much you have learned and remembered. Pain control is an important part of clinical practice so it is important that you understand the action of the various anaesthetics and analgesics.

The answers to these questions are at the end of the book on page 285.

1 What is the usual clinical definition of pain?

2 We generally divide pain into two types: *nociceptive* and ....

3 Another way that pain can be categorised is into *acute* and ....

4 What kind of stimuli would activate nociceptive neurons?

5 Describe the route of a painful stimulus to (say) a finger.

6 What is the function of opioid-like peptides?

7 Name the five key symptoms of inflammation.

8 What is the role of histamine in inflammation?

9 Outline the pathway that results in the synthesis of prostaglandins and thromboxanes.

10 The synthesis of prostaglandins and thromboxanes depends on a cyclo-oxygenase enzyme that exists in at least two forms. Which form is involved in inflammation?

11 What is the role of prostaglandin E_2 in inflammation?

12 Why might an NSAID cause the side-effect of gastro-intestinal bleeding?

13 Why is overdosing with *paracetamol* dangerous?

14 List five common side-effects of opioid drugs.

15 How do local anaesthetics such as *lidocaine* prevent pain during minor surgical procedures?

Answers to questions on page 140

1 Peripheral nervous system.
2 Afferent neurons carry information into the central nervous system.
3 A neuron is a single nerve cell whereas a nerve is a collection of neurons protected by a sheath of connective tissue.
4 The sympathetic and parasympathetic divisions.
5 Skeletal muscles.

Chapter 7

Disorders and drugs of the digestive system

AIMS

By the time you have finished the chapter you should be able to understand:

1 The **physiology** – the structure and function of the digestive system.
2 The **pathology** – those disorders and pathologies associated with the digestive system.
3 The **pharmacology** – the action of the major drug groups used in the treatment of digestive disorders and pathologies.

CONTENTS

The chapter contains some brief case studies and finishes off with self-test questions so you can make sure you have understood the physiology of the digestive system, associated disorders and the pharmacology of drugs used to treat those disorders.

IN PRACTICE

Whatever your branch of clinical practice, you will encounter patients with digestive problems. Sometimes digestive disorders will be the prime reason for them seeking treatment while other patients regard problems such as indigestion, heartburn or constipation as normal and would self-medicate with over-the-counter proprietary medicines. Frequently, digestive problems are **iatrogenic** – a direct consequence of treatment. Examples would be nausea caused by drugs or constipation caused by prolonged stays in hospital. Whatever, their cause, digestive disorders are very common and this is why you need to understand the processes of digestion, the nature of common disorders and the drugs available to treat them.

Iatrogenic is when a patient suffers adverse consequences from treatment. This could be a hospital-acquired infection such as MRSA or adverse reactions from a clinical procedure or drug.

Introduction

Have you ever regretted eating that second helping of pudding? Have you ever thought the hygiene of the fast-food restaurant may have left something to be desired as next day you keep paying frequent visits to the loo? Perhaps a change in diet on holiday left you feeling bloated and less regular than normal? We have all experienced these problems occasionally and may well have used some over-the-counter (OTC) medications such as **indigestion** tablets or **laxatives** to help to ease the symptoms. While unpleasant, generally these problems of the gastro-intestinal tract are temporary and not serious. Within a few hours or days they resolve themselves and we are back to normal. For this reason in this chapter, some problems such as indigestion, **constipation** and **diarrhoea** are being referred to as disorders rather than pathologies. Some disorders, of course, can develop into something more serious, truly deserving of the term pathology. Diarrhoea, for example, can have many causes and mostly the problem is just mildly irritating but sometimes, especially in the very young or very elderly, it can be a life-threatening crisis requiring hospitalisation and IV fluid replacement. **Heartburn** can affect most people occasionally and most sufferers would regard it as a minor problem that can be alleviated with a proprietary **antacid** from the local pharmacy, but it can occasionally develop into more serious **ulcerative oesophagitis.** Those problems truly deserving of the pathology title such as **peptic ulcers, ulcerative colitis** and **Crohn's disease** generally require specialist treatment and although some of the drugs mentioned later in the chapter are part of the treatment regime, detailed discussion of their use is beyond the remit of this introductory book.

WHERE ARE WE STARTING FROM?

In this chapter we shall examine the digestive system in relation to the common disorders that can affect most of us – indigestion, constipation, etc. Most of us will be familiar with the basic structure and function of the digestive system but let's start off with the usual short quiz to find out how much you know before we begin.

1 What is the name of the muscular tube that transfers food from the mouth to the stomach?

   _____

2 What organ secretes digestive enzymes into the duodenum?

   _____

3 What is the large organ that produces bile?

   _____

4 Proteins are important nutrients and the digestive system breaks them down into their component parts called . . .

   _____

5 Would semi-digested food leaving the stomach first encounter the large or small intestine?

   _____

Answers are at the end of the chapter on page 180.

How did you do? If you got all five correct then you will find this chapter relatively straightforward. If you struggled with these questions then it might be an idea to refresh your knowledge of the system from your physiology book – even though we cover the basics in the beginning of this chapter.

7.1 The physiology of the digestive system

The principle task of the digestive system is to transfer the nutrients from the food we eat into our body where those nutrients will be used for processes such as energy, protein production and general tissue maintenance. The digestive system is basically a tube that runs from the mouth to the anus (Figure 7.1). During

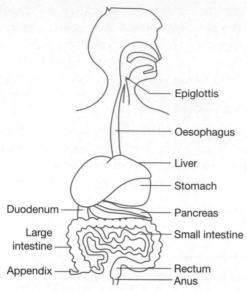

Epiglottis

Oesophagus

Liver

Stomach

Duodenum

Pancreas

Large
intestine

Small intestine

Appendix

Rectum
Anus

Figure 7.1 Layout of the digestive system.

the passage of food along this tube, various chemicals and enzymes are added to break down the food into its component parts. The muscular walls of the gut squash and squeeze the food along the system, which aids the process of breakdown.

There are various accessory organs associated with the digestive system such as the pancreas that secretes a variety of digestive enzymes into the duodenum to assist with the breakdown of food into its component parts. The liver also deserves a mention as it plays a key role in lipid metabolism; it is therefore targeted by drugs such as statins and, as we saw in Chapter 3, the liver plays a key role in drug metabolism. The gall bladder stores the bile produced by the liver and secretes it into the duodenum via the bile duct where it assists in the digestion of lipids.

In Chapter 1 we examined the three main groups of nutrients - carbohydrates, proteins and lipids. We discussed how they need to be in their smallest component parts in order to be suitable for use by our cells. Thus, polysaccharides such as starch need to be broken down into monosaccharides such as glucose, and the proteins need to be disassembled into their component amino acids. Lipid digestion is quite complex but most are broken down into fatty acid molecules that eventually find their way into the bloodstream via the lymphatic system. This is the prime role of the digestive system; to make unpromising chunks of organic matter such as pizza, sausages, salad and chips into molecules small enough to be absorbed from the gut into the body (Figure 7.2).

KEY FACT

The digestive system contributes to homeostasis by maintaining the supply of essential nutrients to the body.

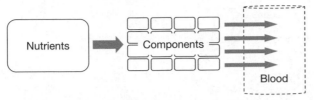

Figure 7.2 Nutrients are broken down in the digestive system into their main component parts that can then be absorbed into the bloodstream and transported to the cells of the body.

The first stage of the digestive process starts in the mouth. Teeth accomplish mechanical digestion by **mastication** (chewing) and chemical digestion is achieved by **saliva** produced by salivary glands. As food is passed to the back of the mouth it triggers the **swallowing reflex**.

Saliva, produced by salivary glands in response to the taste and smell of food, has several functions. It begins the digestion of carbohydrates by the enzyme **amylase** that breaks down polysaccharide starches into more simple sugars – disaccharides and monosaccharides. Saliva also moistens food, allowing it to be swallowed. Antibacterial enzymes in saliva keep the mouth clean and kill bacteria present on food. Saliva also rinses away food debris that may serve as a nutrient source for bacteria.

IN PRACTICE

Any diseases or drugs that inhibit the production of saliva can result in recurrent mouth infections. AIDS patients and those receiving chemotherapy for cancer are at particular risk.

After chewing, food is swallowed and passes down the oesophagus by a ripple of muscular activity called **peristalsis**. At the junction of the oesophagus and **trachea**, a small flap of cartilage called the **epiglottis** prevents food and drink entering the lungs.

Peristalsis explains how you can swallow food even when hanging upside down. The muscles surrounding the digestive tract contract sequentially like a Mexican wave that pushes the food along (even defying gravity).

The stomach is basically a large, muscular bag that stores food before releasing it gradually into the duodenum and small intestine at a rate appropriate for optimal digestion and absorption (Figure 7.3). Muscular contractions by the stomach help to break down food mechanically, while **hydrochloric acid** (HCl) and the enzyme **pepsin** start to break down proteins chemically. The lining of the stomach, the **gastric mucosa**, is protected from its own acid digestive juices

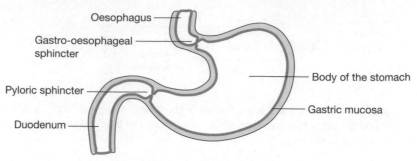

Figure 7.3 Cross-sectional diagram of the stomach.

by a layer of mucus that is produced by secretory cells. The **gastro-oesophageal sphincter** (also called the **cardiac sphincter**) at the entrance of the stomach prevents regurgitation into the oesophagus and the **pyloric** sphincter between the stomach and the duodenum controls the passage of food between the two regions. Sphincters are bands of muscle cells that contract to form a kind of one-way valve. The acidic pulp that empties from the stomach into the duodenum is called **chyme**.

IN PRACTICE

The lumen of the stomach is generally free of bacteria because they are killed by the acidity of pH 2–3. However, one bacterium, *Helicobacter pylori*, seems to thrive at this high level of acidity. *H. pylori* was originally thought of as relatively harmless, but is now known to be one of the main causes of peptic ulcers.

In order to understand the mechanism of certain key drug groups discussed later in Section 7.3, it is necessary to explain the mechanism whereby the gastric mucosa produces hydrochloric acid (HCl).

Hydrochloric acid is made up of hydrogen ions (H^+) and chloride ions (Cl^-). These are secreted separately by the parietal cells of the gastric mucosa and form HCl in the lumen of the stomach:

$$H^+ + Cl^- \rightarrow HCl$$

Note that as the positive charge on the hydrogen ion is cancelled out by the negative charge on the chloride ion, HCl is written without a charge symbol. The hydrogen ion is quite important because its concentration in a solution determines the acidity of that solution. The hydrogen ion is in fact the H in pH and the more hydrogen ions there are, the more acidic is the solution. A hydrogen ion is also effectively a proton. In Chapter 2 we discussed ions and found that they are (usually) atoms that have gained or lost a negatively charged electron. Figure 7.4 shows the structure of a hydrogen atom, consisting of one positively charged proton and one negatively charged electron.

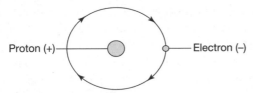

Figure 7.4 A hydrogen atom showing the relationship of the proton and electron (not to scale).

The hydrogen ion is a hydrogen atom that has donated its electron so that there only remains a naked, positively charged proton, i.e. a hydrogen ion. The hydrogen ions are actively pumped by the **parietal** cells of the gastric mucosa into the lumen of the stomach via a proton pump driven by ATP. The movement of positively charged ions into the lumen pulls the negatively charged chloride ions in the same direction, into the lumen of the stomach where they combine to form hydrochloric acid. The parasympathetic nervous system stimulates digestion by increasing the release of HCl and pepsin, especially after the consumption of food. Receptors on the secretory cells of the mucosa are stimulated by acetylcholine released by parasympathetic neurons, the hormone **gastrin** and histamine released by adjacent mast cells (Figure 7.5).

> **KEY FACT**
>
> The secretion of pepsin and HCl is stimulated by histamine, the hormone gastrin and the parasympathetic nervous system releasing acetylcholine.

Moving on from the stomach we come to the duodenum and the pancreas – an important accessory digestive organ that secretes a variety of enzymes, including **amylase**, **proteases** and **lipase** into the duodenum. Amylase breaks

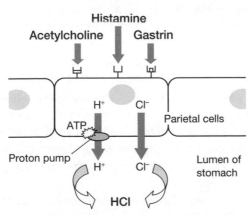

Figure 7.5 The release of hydrochloric acid by the parietal cells is promoted by acetylcholine, histamine and gastrin.

down starch into simple sugars and proteases break down proteins into amino acids. Lipases break down fats with the aid of bile, secreted by the liver, stored in the gallbladder and then released into the duodenum. Alkaline **bicarbonate** is also secreted by the **pancreas** to neutralise the acid chyme and provide a pH more suitable for the pancreatic enzymes. The pancreas also has an endocrine function, secreting the hormones **insulin** and **glucagon** that regulate blood glucose.

> **Insulin** and **glucagon** are released by the pancreas to regulate blood glucose. High blood glucose causes insulin to be released, whereas glucagon is released when blood glucose is low. Insulin lowers blood glucose by stimulating cells to take it in from the blood. Glucagon causes the liver to release stored glucose into the blood.

The small intestine consists of the duodenum, **jejunum** and **ileum.** It is the part of the digestive system where most food is broken down into its basic component parts then absorbed into the bloodstream for distribution to the tissues and cells of the body. The walls of the small intestine contain many folds and projections that increase its surface area in order to optimise the absorption of nutrients (the larger the surface area, the faster the rate of absorption). From the small intestine the remaining undigested material passes into the **caecum** and the **colon** or large intestine.

> **DID YOU KNOW . . .** that the folds and projections inside the small intestine increase its surface area over 500 times – compared to a smooth-walled tube? The length of the small intestine is around 6 metres but without the folds and projections it would need to be around 3 kilometres in length (which would not do much for your waistline).

The main function of the large intestine is the processing and storage of faecal matter, prior to its ejection from the body. The essentially liquid material that enters the colon is transformed into more solid faeces via water reabsorption. Little nutrient absorption occurs in the large intestine except for some vitamins, including vitamin K produced by the gut bacteria and important in blood clotting. Faeces are predominantly water (75%), the remainder being the indigestible components of food, bacteria and cells sloughed from the wall of the digestive tract.

The faeces are expelled by downward pressure on abdominal muscles, generally in response to the **defecation reflex,** triggered by faeces congregating at the end of the colon and stimulating stretch receptors.

A QUICK RECAP on the physiology of the digestive system

- The principle function of the digestive system is to break down food into its component parts that can be easily absorbed into the blood for distribution to the cells of the body.

- Starches are broken down into simple sugars, lipids into fatty acids and proteins into amino acids. The breakdown of food is done chemically and mechanically.

- Accessory organs such as the liver and pancreas secrete enzymes and other chemicals into the digestive tract to help to break down food.

- Most absorption takes place in the small intestine consisting of the duodenum, the jejunum and the ileum.

- Faecal matter in the large intestine is mainly undigested food, bacteria and cells from the lining of the digestive tract.

- Water is absorbed as the faeces move through the large intestine along with some vitamin K produced by resident bacteria.

7.2 Disorders of the digestive system

Diseases can affect any part of the digestive system from the mouth to the anus, and although some can be serious, many common problems such as indigestion, heartburn, diarrhoea and constipation are relatively minor but unpleasant enough to detract from our enjoyment of life.

Disorders of the upper digestive system

Stomach problems are often of uncertain origin and symptoms can be rather vague in nature, including discomfort, bloating, pain and nausea. Common names for these problems include indigestion and heartburn, which are referred to clinically as **dyspepsia** and **gastro-oesophageal reflux**. Before resorting to drugs to manage stomach problems it is generally recommended that lifestyle changes be tried such as reducing alcohol consumption, dietary modification to avoid aggravating foods, weight reduction and giving up smoking. **Gastro-oesophageal reflux disease** (GORD) affects nearly everyone at some time and is caused by stomach acid leaking back through the gastro-oesophageal sphincter into the oesophagus and causing inflammation and pain. Remember that the stomach has a structure that enables it to withstand acid but the oesophagus does not have this protection, so if acid is regurgitated then this can cause damage, inflammation and pain. Symptoms may be worsened by coughing, lifting or by certain foods. Generally, dyspepsia and GORD are temporary problems, but as they can become chronic and perhaps indicate a more serious underlying pathology, persistent symptoms may need further clinical investigation.

171

Peptic ulcers can occur in both the stomach and the duodenum. They are caused by erosion of the gastric mucosa that exposes the underlying tissue to the corrosive influence of stomach acid. Many years ago, stress and spicy foods were considered the main causes of peptic ulcers, but we now know that the bacterium *Helicobacter pylori* is responsible for over 70 per cent of cases. Non-steroidal anti-inflammatory drugs (NSAIDs) discussed in Chapter 6 also contribute to the problem. Symptoms include pain, vomiting, a reduction in appetite and weight loss.

CASE STUDY

Wendy is complaining of abdominal pains and nausea that have been getting worse over the past few weeks. She already suffers from rheumatoid arthritis and regularly takes OTC *ibuprofen* in addition to the antirheumatoid medicines prescribed by her GP. She buys her analgesics from the supermarket as they are cheaper than the chemist. What would you advise?

Comment on case study There is a possibility that *ibuprofen* may be causing the beginning of a peptic ulcer, if Wendy has been taking it regularly for a long time. Self-medication with over-the-counter (OTC) drugs is not always advisable – especially with a long-term problem. If Wendy bought her analgesics from the chemist shop that dispenses her GP-prescribed medicine, the pharmacist would check for side-effects or interactions. Wendy should consult her GP for a check-up and a review of her medication. There are analgesics such as *paracetamol* that may help with the pain without causing stomach problems.

Disorders of the lower digestive system

We now move to the other end of the digestive system and discuss two problems that will have affected nearly everyone at sometime in their lives – diarrhoea and constipation.

Diarrhoea is the frequent passage of liquid faeces and can range from minor discomfort to an emergency requiring fluid and electrolyte replacement. **Acute diarrhoea** can have several causes, including food poisoning that results in **gastroenteritis**, infection of the gastro-intestinal tract. This infection can be caused by bacterial pathogens such as *Campylobacter*, *Salmonella* and *Escherichia* and viral pathogens including **norovirus, astrovirus, adenovirus** and **rotavirus**. **Chronic diarrhoea** has many causes including **irritable bowel syndrome** (IBS), inflammation of the bowel, **Crohn's disease, diverticular disease** and intolerance to foods such as milk (**lactose intolerance**) and wheat (**coeliac disease**).

In the large intestine there is much reabsorption of water along its length, so that by the time they are ready to be excreted, faeces should be reasonably (but not too) firm. Diarrhoea interferes with the normal processing of faecal matter by either increasing motility, resulting in insufficient time for absorption, increasing fluid secretion into the gut, or reducing fluid absorption from the gut (Figure 7.6).

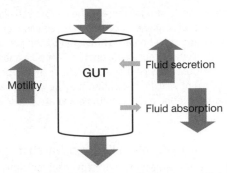

Figure 7.6 Mechanisms that can result in diarrhoea – an increase in motility or fluid secretion or a reduction in fluid absorption.

Constipation is difficult or infrequent defecation that can have many causes, generally a reduction in motility or excessively hard faeces that may be caused by dehydration. Retention can be a problem where, for some reason, people are reluctant to defecate, perhaps finding it painful with haemorrhoids or after abdominal surgery. Dietary causes of constipation are common, especially due to lack of fibre, the indigestible cellulose part of plants. Lack of exercise and various drugs such as opiates and some antidepressants can inhibit gut motility, which reduces the frequency of defecation.

IN PRACTICE

Constipation is very common in hospitals because the patient's mobility is restricted, their diet may be different from normal and pre-operative fluid restriction can add to the problem. Many drugs can cause constipation as a side-effect. Opioids, calcium channel blockers and many anticholinergic drugs all interfere with gut motility.

Haemorrhoids (piles) are enlarged and engorged blood vessels in or around the anus. They are a common and painful problem that affects most of us at some time in our lives. Generally they arise as a result of constipation, pregnancy or inactivity. Symptoms include pain on defecation, bright blood streaked stools and itching. Piles are unpleasant but in themselves not serious and generally they clear up within a week or so, especially if constipation, a common cause, can be resolved.

CASE STUDY

Andy visits Jenny the practice nurse at her weekly surgery. He has been suffering from depression for several months and is now complaining of chronic constipation. Andy's diet appears to be acceptable but you notice that the antidepressant drug he has been prescribed, *amitriptyline*, has anticholinergic effects. Could this be contributing to the problem?

Comment on case study As the name suggests, drugs with anticholinergic activity inhibit the action of acetylcholine, either blocking acetylcholine receptors or reducing general parasympathetic activity. As digestive motility and secretion are stimulated by the parasympathetic nervous system, anticholinergic drugs are likely to cause constipation. Tricyclic antidepressants such as *amitriptyline* have constipation listed as a common side-effect. If the problem does not respond to life-style changes, a review of Andy's medication may be needed. More recent antidepressants such as *fluoxetine* and *paroxetine* may be suitable and are less likely to cause constipation.

Irritable bowel syndrome (IBS) is a relatively mild problem characterised by abdominal pain and discomfort, accompanied by constipation or diarrhoea, but no observable abnormalities show up in tests such as **colonoscopy**. The problem remains enigmatic in its origins which may not have a single cause. Food intolerance, stress and immune dysfunction have all been implicated. This problem should not be confused with **inflammatory bowel syndrome**, which includes Crohn's disease and ulcerative colitis. This is a serious problem that causes ulceration and inflammation in the lower digestive tract and, in extreme cases, perforation of the bowel wall resulting in a clinical emergency. **Antibiotic-associated colitis** is caused by the bacterium *Clostridium difficile* that flourishes after antibacterial drugs have killed off its more susceptible competitors.

> **Colonoscopy** is a procedure to examine the large intestine for signs of disease. After an enema to clear the bowel, a catheter with a spotlight and small video camera linked to a display screen is introduced into the colon.

A QUICK RECAP on disorders of the digestive system

- Dyspepsia and gastro-oesophageal reflux (indigestion and heartburn) are very common problems affecting the upper digestive tract.

- Diarrhoea is another common problem that can be *acute*, often caused by food poisoning, or *chronic*, from problems such as food intolerance or irritable bowel syndrome.

- Constipation can be caused by diet, dehydration, inactivity or drugs such as opiates.

- Haemorrhoids generally have constipation as their cause.

- Irritable bowel syndrome is a relatively common problem whose cause is poorly understood.

- Inflammatory bowel syndrome can be a serious problem resulting in inflammation and ulceration of the colon.

7.3 Drugs used in the management of digestive system disorders

Drugs used in the treatment of mild gastro-oesophageal reflux disease and dyspepsia are similar especially the **antacids** and **alginates**. See the current BNF for recommendations as to which drug should be used for which problem.

> **KEY FACT**
>
> Most drugs that treat gastro-oesophageal reflux disease and dyspepsia aim to reduce the acidity of the stomach contents.

Antacids

Antacids usually contain aluminium or magnesium compounds which, being alkaline, increase the pH of stomach chyme, making it less acid and reducing its irritating effect on the oesophagus. Alginates, extracted from seaweed, form a raft that floats on top of the stomach contents; it reduces reflux and protects the oesophagus from the stomach acid. They are usually combined with an alkaline antacid. Most of these preparations can be obtained without prescription and their brand names such as Acidex® and Gaviscon® may already be familiar to you.

H$_2$ receptor antagonists

This group of drugs are used to treat GORD, peptic and duodenal ulcers. Examples include *cimetidine, famotidine, nizatidine* and *ranitidine*.

As the name implies, these drugs work by blocking **H$_2$ receptors** in the gastric mucosa. As we saw earlier in the chapter, gastric secretions are stimulated by various chemical messengers – including histamine. Histamine binds to the H$_2$ sub-class of histamine receptors on the parietal cells of the gastric mucosa and stimulates the release of hydrochloric acid (HCl). H$_2$ receptor antagonists work by blocking the H$_2$ receptors from the stimulatory effect of histamine and thus reduce the secretion of hydrochloric acid (Figure 7.7). The stomach contents become less acidic which relieves the symptoms of discomfort.

> **IN PRACTICE**
>
> *Cimetidine* especially can interact with other drugs by inhibiting P450 cytochrome enzymes in the liver (see Chapter 3). These enzymes break down various substances, including drugs, and blocking their action can increase the serum levels of drugs such as *warfarin, phenytoin* and *aminophylline*.

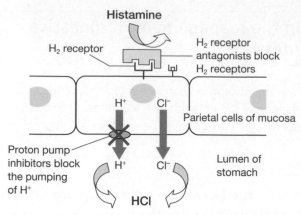

Figure 7.7 Showing how H$_2$ receptor antagonists and proton-pump inhibitors reduce the secretion of hydrochloric acid from the parietal cells of the mucosa into the lumen of the stomach.

Proton-pump inhibitors

This group of drugs is used for the treatment of peptic ulcers, dyspepsia and GORD. They are also indicated for use with antibacterial drugs in the eradication of *Helicobacter pylori*. Examples of the group include; **esomeprazole, lansoprazole, omeprazole, pantoprazole** and **rabeprazole**.

These drugs work by irreversibly inhibiting the proton pump in the parietal cells of the mucosa, thus preventing hydrogen ions being pumped into the lumen of the stomach, and slowing the formation of hydrochloric acid (Figure 7.7). **Proton-pump inhibitors** selectively accumulate in the parietal cells of the mucosa, and despite having a relatively short half-life can exert their effect for several days.

DID YOU KNOW . . . that there has been interest recently in the beneficial effects of proton-pump inhibitors in asthma sufferers? It was discovered by chance that when being treated for digestive problems with PPIs, some asthmatics appeared to experience an improvement in their asthma symptoms. The mechanism whereby this happens is not yet understood.

Drugs used in the treatment of diarrhoea

In developed countries, acute diarrhoea is unpleasant but not generally life-threatening, although neonates and the elderly may be at particular risk. In severe cases, rehydration can be required but generally the problem resolves itself in a few days. Except in cases of serious bacterial infection, it is not generally recommended that antibacterial drugs are prescribed for diarrhoea. This is because it can be difficult to determine if the problem is indeed bacterial in origin, and most cases are self-limiting. If the cause of diarrhoea is viral, no suitable antiviral drugs are available. Antimotility drugs can be used in cases of uncomplicated acute diarrhoea but are not recommended for young children.

Antimotility drugs are mainly based on drugs that have constipation as a side-effect and include **codeine phosphate**, **co-phenotrope**, **loperamide hydrochloride** and **morphine**. Opiates are well known for causing constipation by reducing gut motility and so this allows more time for the gut to reabsorb water, making the faeces less liquid and reducing the frequency of evacuation.

Some of the preparations mentioned above are combination drugs. **Co-phenotrope** is a combination of the opiate **diphenoxylate** and the anticholinergic drug **atropine**. **Morphine** is generally combined with **kaolin**, a type of clay that holds moisture and increases the viscosity of the gut contents.

Drugs and preparations used in the treatment of constipation

Constipation is often associated with lifestyle or pathologies not directly related to the gastro-intestinal system. Treatment therefore is usually first directed at lifestyle changes where possible. Exercise, adequate fluid intake and a diet containing plenty of fresh fruit, vegetables and fibre-containing cereals are a formula for keeping the bowels regular and avoiding constipation. Many drugs such as opioids and antidepressants are well known causes of constipation but it may not be practical or safe to change medication in the short term. Haemorrhoids make defecation painful, encouraging retention of faeces, so treating the haemorrhoids may relieve the constipation. Where pharmacological treatment is the only option to relieve constipation, there are three classes of **laxatives**:

- **Bulk forming laxatives** - these are preparations high in insoluble plant cellulose. They increase the faecal mass and stimulate peristalsis. Examples include **ispaghula husk**, **methylcellulose** and **sterculia**.

- **Osmotic laxatives** - these modify the osmotic environment and pull water into the colon which softens stools and increases faecal mass. Examples include **lactulose** and **macrogols** (polyethylene glycols).

- **Stimulant laxatives** - these increase fluid secretion into the gut, softening the stools and also stimulating peristalsis. Examples include **bisacodyl**, **docusate** and **senna**.

Drugs and preparations used in the treatment of haemorrhoids (piles)

As constipation is a common cause of haemorrhoids, the first line of treatment may be to treat the constipation, either with lifestyle changes or the drugs and preparations mentioned above. Preparations for haemorrhoids are generally designed to reduce inflammation, pain and itching. They are sold in combination preparations that may contain anti-inflammatory steroids such as *hydrocortisone*, local anaesthetics such as *lidocaine* and mild astringents such as *zinc oxide*. All may be combined into ointment or suppositories.

Drugs used in the treatment of irritable bowel syndrome

Irritable bowel syndrome is usually managed by a variety of lifestyle modifications before resorting to drugs. Changes in diet often help with the problem but failing that, antimuscarinic drugs such as *atropine sulphate* that reduce gut motility by inhibiting parasympathetic activity can be used. *Alvarine*, *mebeverine* and *peppermint oil* are also used to relieve abdominal colic and distension in IBS but their mechanism of action is uncertain.

A QUICK RECAP on drugs used in the management of digestive system disorders

- Dyspepsia and gastro-oesophageal reflux are generally treated with drugs that reduce stomach acid, either by neutralising it with alkaline preparations or inhibiting its secretion.

- Drugs that inhibit the secretion of stomach acid include H_2 receptor antagonists such as *cimetidine* and proton pump inhibitors such as *omeprazole*.

- Drugs used to treat diarrhoea are generally based on opioids that cause constipation as, in this case, a useful side-effect.

- Constipation is primarily treated with adjustments to lifestyle but bulk-forming, osmotic and stimulant laxatives may be useful.

- Haemorrhoids are treated with combination compounds of anti-inflammatory steroids, local anaesthetics and mild astringents.

- Treatment of IBS usually involves drugs such as *atropine* that reduces gut motility and therefore spasm induced pain.

RUNNING WORDS

Here are some of the technical terms that were included in this chapter. Read through them one by one and tick them off when you are sure that you understand them.

Acute diarrhoea p. 172
Adenovirus p. 172
Alginates p. 175
Amylase p. 167
Antacid p. 164
Antibiotic-associated colitis p. 174
Astrovirus p. 172
Bicarbonate p. 170
Bulk-forming laxatives p. 177
Caecum p. 170
Campylobacter p. 172
Cardiac sphincter p. 168
Chronic diarrhoea p. 172
Chyme p. 168
Coeliac disease p. 172
Colon p. 170
Colonoscopy p. 174
Constipation p. 164
Crohn's disease p. 164
Defecation reflex p. 170
Diarrhoea p. 164
Diverticular disease p. 172
Dyspepsia p. 170

Epiglottis p. 167
Escherichia p. 172
Gastric mucosa p. 167
Gastrin p. 169
Gastroenteritis p. 172
Gastro-oesophageal reflux disease (GORD) p. 170
Gastro-oesophageal sphincter p. 168
Glucagon p. 170
H_2 receptors p. 175
Haemorrhoids p. 173
Heartburn p. 164
Hydrochloric acid p. 167
Iatrogenic p. 164
Ileum p. 170
Indigestion p. 164
Inflammatory bowel syndrome p. 174
Insulin p. 170
Irritable bowel syndrome p. 172
Jejunum p. 170
Lactose intolerance p. 172

Laxatives p. 164
Lipase p. 169
Mastication p. 167
Norovirus p. 172
Osmotic laxatives p. 177
Pancreas p. 170
Parietal p. 169
Pepsin p. 167
Peptic ulcers p. 164
Peristalsis p. 167
Proteases p. 169
Proton-pump inhibitors p. 176
Pyloric sphincter p. 168
Rotavirus p. 172
Saliva p. 167
Salmonella p. 172
Stimulant laxatives p. 177
Swallowing reflex p. 167
Trachea p. 167
Ulcerative colitis p. 164
Ulcerative oesophagitis p. 164

REFERENCES AND FURTHER RECOMMENDED READING

All recommended websites are open access (but free registration is sometimes required).

Bandolier: gastroenterology – http://www.medicine.ox.ac.uk/bandolier/

NHS Website – http://www.nhs.uk/Conditions/

Your turn to try

Now you have finished reading through this chapter try answering these questions to see how much you have learned.

The answers to these questions are at the end of the book on page 286.

1 Name the three sections of the small intestine.

2 Proteins are broken down into their component parts called ....

3 What is the enzyme in saliva that breaks down starches?

4 Name the two sphincters in the stomach.

5 Name the digestive enzyme secreted into the stomach that denatures proteins.

6 Name three chemical messengers that stimulate the release of hydrochloric acid.

7 Which organ secretes digestive enzymes into the duodenum?

8 Heartburn is the commonly used name for what disorder?

9 Which bacterium is responsible for most cases of peptic ulcer?

10 Would a reduction in motility in the large intestine be most likely to cause constipation or diarrhoea?

11 How do alginates help to reduce the symptoms of gastro-oesophageal reflux?

12 What type of receptor is targeted by *cimetidine*?

13 How do proton-pump inhibitors reduce stomach acid?

14 A side-effect of which group of drugs is useful in the treatment of diarrhoea?

15 How do osmotic laxatives work?

Answers to questions on page 165

1 The oesophagus.
2 The pancreas.
3 The liver.
4 Amino acids.
5 The small intestine.

Chapter 8

Infection and antimicrobial drugs (bugs and drugs)

AIMS

By the time you have finished the chapter you should be able to understand:

1 The **nature of microbes** – basic microbiology.
2 The **classification of microbes** – the different groups, especially the pathogens.
3 The **pathology** – the diseases caused by microbes.
4 The **pharmacology** – the action of the major drug groups used against microbial infection.

CONTENTS

The chapter contains some brief case studies and finishes off with self-test questions to enable you to make sure that you have understood the nature of microbes, associated disorders and the pharmacology of antimicrobial drugs.

IN PRACTICE

Drugs that treat microbial infections are extensively used in most areas of clinical practice, both in primary care and the hospital setting. In primary care, infections are very common and you will encounter patients with coughs, colds, sore throats, flu, cystitis and numerous other unpleasant but rarely fatal diseases – except perhaps in vulnerable patients such as the elderly. In hospitals, staff not only treat patients with infectious diseases but also put considerable effort into preventing uninfected patients from contracting diseases. This means that you may well find yourself in an area of clinical practice where your patients have contracted an infection or are vulnerable to contracting infections. It is important, therefore, that you have a good understanding of the nature of the various pathogenic microorganisms, the diseases they cause and how the drugs work that we use to treat microbial infections.

Introduction

Everyone reading this will undoubtedly have suffered from a **bacterial**, **viral** or **fungal** infection at some time in their lives. In our environment, we are surrounded by innumerable small organisms, collectively called **microbes**. Although most of them are perfectly harmless, some cause disease and in our crowded world it is very easy to pick up infections. Different microbes cause different diseases, so if you have had a cold then it was caused by a virus, probably **rhinovirus** that affects the upper respiratory tract (not the large African animal with a horn on its head). If you have had a sore throat, then that may have been a bacterial infection caused by *Streptococcus*. **Candidiasis**, commonly called **thrush**, will have been caused by a fungus called *Candida albicans*. All of these organisms can cause disease in humans but they are very different from each other. A bacterium is as different from a fungus or virus as we are from a dandelion. This means that the methods whereby they cause disease are different and, very importantly, the drugs that we use to combat them are very different. So, to understand antimicrobial pharmacology you really need to know something about the microbes themselves. You need to understand their structure, how they reproduce, how they are spread and how they cause infection.

Another important feature that will be covered in this chapter is how microbes, especially bacteria, can develop resistance to antimicrobial drugs. Hospital infections are constantly in the news, especially those caused by organisms such as meticillin resistant *Staphylococcus aureus* (MRSA) and *Clostridium difficile*. These organisms are causing real problems because they quickly develop resistance to new antibacterial drugs and the use of these drugs is now much more carefully controlled in an attempt to prevent resistant strains developing and spreading.

Antimicrobial drugs are widely used in hospitals and primary care, so it is important that you understand how they work and why they must be used with caution.

> **Antimicrobial (drug)** refers to any drug that is targeted at a microbe. Drugs targeted at specific groups of microbes now have specific names, thus we have antibacterial drugs, antiviral drugs, antifungal drugs, etc. The term 'antibiotic' is used less often these days.

We are going to subdivide the microbes into their various groups, but first let us define our terms. Microbes, or **microorganisms**, are very small organisms that can only be seen using a microscope. There are many types of microbes but most of them that cause disease belong to the following groups:

- Bacteria
- Fungi
- Viruses
- Protozoa

There are also other small, parasitic organisms such as **helminths** (worms) that cause disease, but whether these truly fit into the category of microbes is open to debate. From a pharmacological view, these organisms cause infections, and as they appear in the same section of the BNF as bacteria, fungi and viruses, we will include them in this chapter.

WHERE ARE WE STARTING FROM?

In this chapter we will be exploring the wonderful world of germs, how they cause disease and finally, how we thwart their plans with antimicrobial drugs. Even if you have a reasonable knowledge of human physiology, it may be that you have not studied microbial physiology, so we will start with our usual short quiz to see what you know.

1 Is *Candida albicans* (the organism that causes thrush) a bacterium, a fungus or a virus?

_____

2 What does MRSA stand for?

_____

3 Which organism is the bigger: a bacterium or a virus?

_____

4 What type of organism causes the common cold?

_____

5 Can you treat the common cold with penicillin?

_____

Answers are at the end of the chapter on page 205.

How did you do? Don't worry if you struggled because microbiology is not a subject that is taught much outside of universities. However, you need to know the basics in order to understand microbial disease and treatment and the following few pages will provide a good starting point for your studies.

8.1   How do microorganisms fit into the scheme of life?

Antimicrobial drugs target microbial cells but, unfortunately, those cells are found amid the human cells within our bodies. It is therefore important that antimicrobial drugs differentiate microbial cells from human cells – otherwise the human cells will be damaged by the drugs. Fortunately, the structures and proteins that are found within microbial cells make them sufficiently different from human cells and allow us to target them with antimicrobial drugs. Because different groups of microbes have different structures or targets, it is first necessary to establish how the various groups fit into the scheme of life. When we have done this, we can then decide how to deal with them.

All life on the planet appears to reside within one of the five kingdoms of organisms, as shown in Figure 8.1. Bacteria form the oldest kingdom and were one of the first organisms to evolve on Earth, some three billion years ago. It is believed that all other organisms on the planet evolved from bacterial ancestors. Plants, animals, fungi and a kingdom of (mostly) single-celled organisms called **protoctista** evolved more recently, and are much more closely related to each other than they are to bacteria.

That's five kingdoms – what about the viruses?

Good question. Viruses are a problem because there is some disagreement as to whether they can be classified as being alive – or not, let alone them having a kingdom of their own. There is also uncertainty about how they are related to the other five kingdoms.

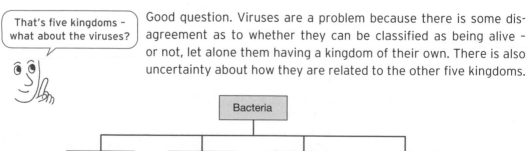

Figure 8.1 All life on Earth can be allocated to one of the five kingdoms.

As well as dividing life between the five kingdoms, there is a more fundamental division between bacteria and other cellular organisms. Bacteria are all single-celled organisms and their cell structure is relatively simple. They do not have a nucleus and are called **prokaryotes**. All other cellular organisms such as plants, animals, fungi and protoctista have more complex cells with nuclei and are called **eukaryotes**. As viruses are not cellular they do not really fit into either category. Let us now examine our five groups of organisms that are responsible for most infectious diseases in humans, starting with bacteria.

> **Prokaryote** – means 'pre-nucleus' (*karyon* being Greek for nucleus). **Eukaryote**-means 'true nucleus'.

8.2 Bacteria

Bacteria are undoubtedly the most successful group of organisms ever to have evolved on planet Earth. The mighty dinosaurs ruled supreme for tens of millions of years but their reign was short compared to the bacteria that emerged from unknown origins over three thousand million years ago and are still with us today. Bacteria make up the greatest biomass on the planet, bigger than all of the rain forests put together. They have adapted to live almost everywhere on the planet, from hot springs to frozen tundra, from the deepest seas to the highest mountains – so it is hardly surprising that our bodies make very pleasant, comfortable homes for them.

Bacteria are small, generally between 1.0 and 2.0 μm (1 μm = 1/1000 mm), which means that they are invisible to the naked eye. They grow rapidly by cell division, one bacterium splits into two, then each of those split into two, and so on – less than 20 minutes for each cell cycle in ideal conditions. Believe it or not, in 12 hours one bacterium could theoretically divide over 36 times and produce around 35 billion new cells. This is why it is dangerous to leave cooked food unrefrigerated overnight because a few hundred bacteria that settled on the food the day before have become trillions of bacteria by the next day. Our digestive enzymes and stomach acid that were quite sufficient to deal with a few hundred bacteria may be overwhelmed by the sheer numbers produced by uncontrolled overnight proliferation. The bacteria pass through the stomach into the small intestine and can cause infection along with the symptoms of food poisoning. Of course, the constant doubling rate described above is seldom encountered outside the laboratory, but even so, given the right conditions, a small colony of bacteria can quickly become a big colony.

So refrigeration doesn't kill bacteria then?

No, low temperatures slow down bacterial metabolism and so reduces the rate at which they multiply. The body's defences can cope with the small numbers of bacteria that we inevitably consume with our food every day.

The structure of bacteria

Bacteria are diverse and come in many different shapes but they all have some common characteristics. Bacteria are single-celled organisms and although some bacteria do form aggregations, each cell is essentially self-sufficient. Also, unlike eukaryotic cells, bacteria do not have membrane-bound organelles such as mitochondria, endoplasmic reticulum, Golgi apparatus or nucleus. Bacteria do have DNA that codes for their proteins but it is not grouped into a nucleus enclosed by a nuclear membrane. The cell wall is another unique feature of bacteria, and this is described shortly in more detail as it is an important target for some drugs.

Some bacteria are **motile** (able to move). While they are not likely to chase you down the street, they can move a few micrometres towards a more promising source of nutrients. This limited locomotion is achieved by means of **flagella**, fine whip-like structures that propel the bacteria along. The **fimbriae**, fine hair-like structures that can be seen on some bacteria, are not used for movement but are believed to be involved with attachment to the host's tissue. Figure 8.2 shows the structure of a typical bacterium.

Some bacteria such as *Clostridium* can undergo a form of hibernation by forming tough outer coats called **endospores**. These dormant structures can survive long periods without water and are highly resistant to our attempts to eradicate them with detergents and disinfectants. This means that rooms and equipment that appear clean can harbour bacterial endospores that can eventually re-emerge into fully functional pathogens that can cause disease.

Most bacteria do not invade human cells and are found in the interstitium or on the epithelial tissue that lines mucus membranes and skin. A few bacteria such as *Chlamydia* are **obligate** intracellular parasites that can only reproduce within their host's cells.

> **Obligate** is a word frequently encountered in microbiology that refers to microbes with very specific nutritional or environmental requirements. Thus obligate intracellular parasites cannot reproduce outside of their host's cells.

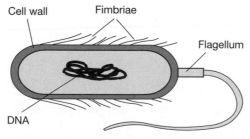

Figure 8.2 Structure of a typical bacterium.

The classification of bacteria

Of all organisms, bacteria are perhaps among the most diverse and difficult to classify. Despite them all being relatively simple, single-celled organisms, they exhibit much variety in their structure and metabolism. If you look in the *British National Formulary* or any other listing of currently available antibacterial drugs, you will see that these drugs tend to target specific groups of bacteria, and as there are specific terms that are used to describe these groups, it is important that you spend a little time understanding basic bacterial classification.

There are a lot of different bacteria in the environment and while most of them are relatively harmless to humans, there are quite a few that are pathogenic, i.e. they have the ability to cause disease. Common pathogenic bacteria and the infections they cause include:

- *Escherichia coli* – diarrhoea, vomiting and cystitis
- *Enterococci species* – bacteraemia, bacterial endocarditis
- *Staphylococcus aureus* – wound infection and septicaemia
- *Salmonella species* – diarrhoea and vomiting
- *Streptococci species* – sore throat, scarlet fever, rheumatic fever, meningitis
- *Helicobacter pylori* – stomach ulcers
- *Pseudomonas aeruginosa* – pneumonia and septicaemia
- *Clostridium difficile* – colitis
- *Campylobacter species* – diarrhoea
- *Chlamydia trachomatis* - sexually transmitted infection
- *Haemophilus influenzae* – pneumonia and bacterial meningitis.

Some of these bacteria are called **opportunist pathogens** because they only cause disease when the opportunity arises, perhaps because someone's immune system has been suppressed, either by illness or immunosuppressive drugs. Otherwise, these bacteria live in and on us as **commensals**, generally without causing any problems. From a clinical view, it is important to know something about the different groups because to some extent, the group that a bacterium belongs to will determine the antibacterial drug chosen to target it. We could spend the whole of this book examining the classification of bacteria but we will limit ourselves to groupings that have relevance to the type of drugs used, starting with the bacterial cell wall.

> **Commensals** are bacteria that live in and on us, benefiting from our body in terms of nutrients but not doing us any harm. They sometimes inadvertently benefit us by out-competing pathogenic bacteria and in the gut may produce useful substances such as vitamin K.

Classification by cell wall

The structure of the bacterial cell wall can influence the type of antibacterial drug used and you will find two broad categories mentioned in the BNF – **Gram positive** and **Gram negative**. **Christian Gram** was a Danish microbiologist (1853–1938) who developed a technique of staining bacteria so that they could be viewed under the optical microscope. Normally, bacteria are colourless and you have to stain them with a chemical pigment such as **crystal violet** in order to see them properly. Gram found that bacteria appeared to be divided into two groups, those that were stained by his staining technique and those that were not. This proved such a useful tool in classifying bacteria that the two groups were named Gram positive and Gram negative in his honour. It was later found that the reason for each group's different reaction to Gram's stain was that their cell wall was significantly different in structure.

The bacterial cell wall contains a substance unique to bacteria called **peptido-glycan**. This is a complex molecule, containing proteins, sugars and acids. Its purpose is to provide integrity and strength to the cell wall of the bacterium. Gram-positive bacteria have a cell wall comprising mainly of peptidoglycan whereas Gram-negative bacteria have a thin layer of peptidoglycan sandwiched between two membranes. Figure 8.3 shows a much simplified depiction of the Gram-positive and Gram-negative bacterial cell wall.

Worthy of mention is a bacterial enzyme called **transpeptidase**. This has a central role in the production of peptidoglycan and it is this enzyme that is targeted by antibacterials such as **penicillins** and **cephalosporins**. The pharmacological relevance of the cell wall structure is that generally, Gram-positive organisms are more resistant to antimicrobial drugs because their cell wall is more complex and this makes drug penetration more difficult.

Gram-positive species include:

- *Enterococci species*
- *Staphylococcus aureus*
- *Streptococci species*
- *Clostridium difficile*

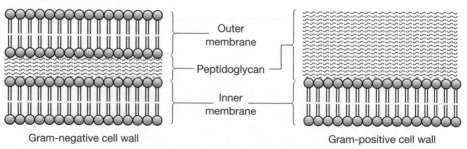

Gram-negative cell wall   Gram-positive cell wall

Figure 8.3 Simplified structure of the Gram-positive and Gram-negative cell wall.

Gram-negative species include:

- *Escherichia coli*
- *Salmonella species*
- *Helicobacter pylori*
- *Pseudomonas aeruginosa*
- *Campylobacter species*
- *Chlamydia trachomatis*
- *Haemophilus influenzae*

Classification by oxygen requirement

You will find that in the BNF, some antibacterial drugs are mentioned as being particularly suitable for **anaerobic** bacteria, so we need a brief exploration of this method of grouping bacteria. Some bacteria such as *Pseudomonas* require oxygen and are called **aerobes**. Others such as *Clostridium* and *Chlamydia* require an oxygen-free environment and are called **anaerobes**. Whether bacteria are aerobes or anaerobes can determine the choice of antibacterial drug.

As is usual with bacteria, they refuse to divide themselves into neat categories and you will come across some of them that are partially aerobic and partially anaerobic. These are the **facultative anaerobes** such as *Pseudomonas*, *Staphylococci* and *Escherichia* that can switch their metabolism depending on whether oxygen is present or not.

Classification by shape

Bacteria come in various shapes and these are used in classification (Figure 8.4). The two largest groups are **bacilli**, which are rod shaped, and **cocci** which are spherical. The cocci can group themselves further by the way that they form aggregations. *Diplococci* tend to form in pairs, *Streptococci* form chains and *Staphylococci* form groups that look rather like bunches of grapes.

How bacteria cause disease

We know that many bacteria are opportunistic pathogens that can multiply when conditions are amenable, but how do they actually cause disease? How is it that

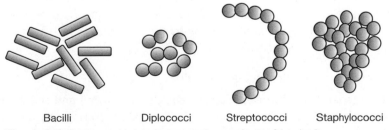

| Bacilli | Diplococci | Streptococci | Staphylococci |

Figure 8.4 Some common shapes and groupings of bacteria.

something as small as bacteria can produce such unpleasant diseases in organisms millions of times their size? Some bacteria such as *Staphylococci*, *Streptococci* and *Clostridium* release toxins, which are chemicals that damage the host cells and their membranes. Other bacteria have components of their cell wall that appear to make the bacterial cell itself intrinsically toxic. These include many Gram-negative genuses such as *Escherichia*, *Pseudomonas* and *Salmonella*. For many bacteria, the precise mechanism whereby they cause disease is not fully understood.

DID YOU KNOW . . . that *staphyle* is Greek for bunch of grapes? *Staphylococci* are so named because they are cocci that aggregate into groups that look rather like bunches of grapes when viewed under the electron microscope.

A QUICK RECAP on bacteria

- Bacteria are single-celled organisms that can reproduce very quickly by cell division.

- Bacteria are prokaryotic organisms meaning that they do not have a true nucleus.

- Bacteria can be classified by their cell wall into Gram-positive and Gram-negative species.

- Bacteria can also be classified by their shape, their motility and their ability to tolerate oxygen.

- Many bacteria live in and on us as commensals but can cause disease when the opportunity arises. These are called opportunistic pathogens.

Antibacterial drugs

In 1928, the Scottish microbiologist, Alexander Fleming, was working at St Mary's hospital in London when he accidentally discovered penicillin, the first effective antibacterial drug. Fleming found that some of his cultures of *Staphylococcus aureus* had been contaminated by the mould *Penicillium notatum* that had killed the bacteria. Unable to manufacture the antibacterial substance produced by the mould in any quantity, Fleming went on to other work but later his discovery was taken up by two other researchers, Howard Florey and Ernst Chain. They successfully produced the antibacterial substance, now named penicillin, in sufficient quantities to save many Allied soldiers' lives in the second part of World War II. In 1945, Fleming, Florey and Chain jointly received the Nobel Prize in Medicine for their discovery of penicillin.

Principles of antibacterial action

Antibacterial drugs target bacterial cells that are living and reproducing within the human body so if these drugs are going to kill bacterial cells and leave human cells unharmed then they will have to target structures that are found in bacterial cells but not in human cells. This is called the principle of **selective toxicity** – where a drug kills the harmful bacteria without damaging the host's cells. Fortunately, humans are eukaryotic and bacteria are prokaryotic so there are quite a few differences that we can identify as targets.

> **KEY FACT**
>
> Antibacterial drugs must target bacterial cell structures that are different from those found in eukaryotic human cells.

Some drugs, the **broad spectrum** antibacterials, are effective against a wide range of bacteria, both Gram-positive and Gram-negative. Other antibacterials, termed **narrow spectrum**, are used against specific families or groups of bacteria.

> **IN PRACTICE**
>
> Broad spectrum antibacterials can be quite useful if a bacterial infection is diagnosed but the type of bacteria that is causing the infection has not been identified. This type of prescribing is sometimes called 'blind therapy'.

Bactericidal and bacteriostatic action

Bacteria can either be killed with a drug that has a **bactericidal** action or their growth inhibited with a drug that has **bacteriostatic** activity. The benefit of killing a bacterial colony is self evident but of inhibiting its growth less so. In the latter scenario, the body's immune system is better able to recognise and destroy a static rather than expanding colony of invading bacteria. Drugs that attack the cell wall have a bactericidal action – and by definition a bacteriostatic action. Drugs that inhibit protein synthesis tend to be more bacteriostatic, although they may also be bactericidal at higher doses.

Antibacterials 1: drugs targeting the cell wall

This group of drugs, sometimes called the **beta-lactams** (β-lactams), comprises the penicillins, cephalosporins and carbapenems which are widely used and contain some of the most commonly prescribed broad spectrum antibacterials. Penicillins include *amoxicillin, ampicillin, benzylpenicillin, phenoxymethylpenicillin, flucloxacillin* and *temocillin*. Cephalosporins include *cefaclor, cefadroxil, cefalexin, cefixime, cefotaxime, cefpodoxime, ceftazidime, ceftriaxone* and *cefuroxime*. Both groups are effective when used for various common bacterial infections such as throat infections, tonsillitis, ear infections and urinary tract infections (UTI) as well as more serious problems such as **septicaemia** (systemic infections), **endocarditis** (heart infections) and **meningitis** (inflammation of the lining of the brain). *Aztreonam*, also a β-lactam, is the sole representative of its group and is effective against

Gram-negative aerobes. The **carbapenems** have a wider spectrum of activity and include *ertapenem*, *imipenem* and *meropenem*.

> ## CASE STUDY
>
> Devinder arrives at your practice with a sick child. Manjit, aged 5, is very ill with the classic symptoms of meningitis – stiff neck, fever, vomiting, headache, etc. His mother says he is allergic to penicillin – what would you do?

Comment on case study Urgent referral to the nearest hospital is required because meningitis can be life threatening. Manjit needs immediate antibacterials so a broad spectrum cephalosporin could overcome the problem of his allergy to penicillins. This should be administered intravenously to hasten its effects. As the child is vomiting, oral antibacterials would not be appropriate.

The penicillins, cephalosporins and carbapenems belong to a group of drugs called **β-lactam** antibacterials as their molecular structure contains a functional group called a **β-lactam ring**. We generally try to avoid too many molecular structures in *Introducing Pharmacology* but as this term is mentioned in the BNF, we need to know what it means. Figure 8.5 shows the basic structure of penicillin and cephalosporin and you will see that they are relatively simple molecules that both contain a β-lactam ring. This ring is of pharmacological importance because, apart from it being essential to penicillin's antibacterial action, it is targeted by bacteria themselves.

A key difference between bacterial and human cells is the bacterial cell wall that contains the structural molecule **peptidoglycan** as one of its key components. Peptidoglycan is unique to bacteria and so it makes a good target as human cells will be unaffected. Bacteria make peptidoglycan with the help of the bacterial enzyme transpeptidase, again unique to bacteria, and it is this enzyme that is targeted by the β-lactam antibacterials. With the inhibition of transpeptidase, bacteria cannot make their cell wall properly so it becomes unstable, causing the bacteria to **lyse** (burst) and die.

> **DID YOU KNOW ...** that penicillin is excreted unchanged in the urine? In its early days, penicillin was so difficult to produce that doctors would collect the patient's urine, extract the penicillin and re-inject it back into the patient.

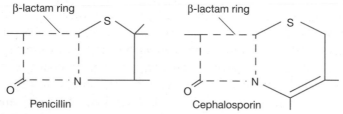

Figure 8.5 Molecular skeleton of penicillin and cephalosporin showing β-lactam ring defined by a hatched line.

Bacterial resistance to the β-lactam antibacterials

Before we discuss the β-lactam antibacterials further, we need to have a brief diversion into **bacterial resistance**. The reason for this is that the choice of antibacterial drug can be determined by whether the target organism is one that has developed resistance – or not.

We tend to think of bacterial resistance as a relatively recent phenomenon. In fact as early as the 1940s, isolated cases of resistance to the early antibacterial drugs had been observed. Strains of *Staphylococcus aureus* were among the first organisms to exhibit resistance, but by the 1980s resistance among pathogenic bacteria was becoming widespread and creating serious problems, especially in hospitals.

Bacteria are prone to genetic mutation and in any population of a particular strain, there are likely to be a few individual bacteria that exhibit resistance to a particular antibacterial drug. Normally, a few resistant bacteria in a population of trillions should not cause problems because their numbers are relatively insignificant. However, what happens when we treat a patient with an antibacterial drug and kill all of the susceptible bacteria, leaving behind only those that are resistant to that drug? When this happens the resistant bacteria can proliferate without the constraint of competition and, because of the speed at which they can multiply, very soon they become the predominant strain (Figure 8.6). Antibacterial drugs are unable to kill them and so the resistant strains can continue to cause disease and spread to other patients, especially those who are already sick and susceptible to infection – as you might find in a hospital.

There are many ways that bacteria can develop resistance but one of the most common mechanisms is for them to produce enzymes that inactivate the antibacterial drugs. Such enzymes are the **β-lactamases**, produced by many resistant bacteria that inactivate β-lactam drugs such as penicillin and cephalosporin. The name of the enzyme group gives us a clue to the action of β-lactamases which target and break the β-lactam ring, rendering the drugs ineffective (Figure 8.7). β-lactamases that have affinity for penicillins and cephalosporins are called **penicillinases** and **cephalosporinases** respectively.

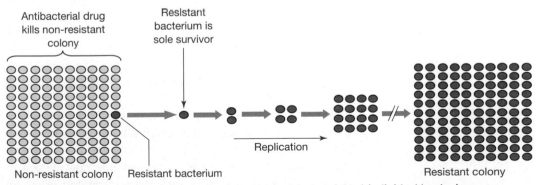

Figure 8.6 How bacterial resistance develops. An isolated resistant individual bacterium can quickly become the dominant strain when an antibacterial drug kills off the remaining bacteria in a non-resistant colony.

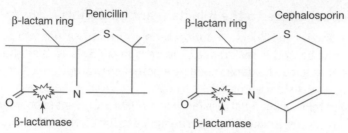

Figure 8.7 Bacterial β-lactamase enzymes attack the β-lactam of penicillins and cephalosporins, rendering them ineffective.

> **Penicillinases** and **cephalosporinases** are enzymes of the **β-lactamase** family that target and denature some penicillins and cephalosporins so rendering them harmless to bacteria.

β-Lactam antibacterials effective against resistant bacteria

Few β-lactam antibacterials are wholly immune from attack by β-lactamase-producing resistant bacteria. *Flucloxacillin* and *temocillin* are not inactivated by most β-lactamases and are thus generally effective against resistant *Staphylococcus* species. Because of the danger of resistance developing to these drugs, their use is reserved for infections caused by existing β-lactamase-resistant strains.

> **IN PRACTICE**
>
> *Meticillin*-resistant *Staphylococcus aureus,* or MRSA as it is popularly called, is a major problem in many hospitals where it can cause post-surgical and other wound infections. *Meticillin* is now discontinued but MRSA continues its march of resistance through the pharmacopoeia and relatively few antibacterial drugs remain effective against it.

Co-amoxiclav is a clever combination of drugs that attempt to overcome bacterial resistance from β-lactamase-producing bacteria. The drug consists of a mixture of *amoxicillin,* an effective (but susceptible to penicillinase) broad spectrum antibacterial and *clavulanic acid.* The latter drug has no antibacterial action but is an effective inhibitor of bacterial β-lactamase. In other words, it binds to and blocks the action of β-lactamase, thus allowing *amoxicillin* to get on with its task of destroying bacteria. If you look at the molecular structure of *clavulanic acid* in Figure 8.8, you will note how close it is to the β-lactam skeleton of *penicillin* and related drugs. It is because of the structural similarity between *penicillin* and *clavulanic acid* that they are both targets for β-lactamase.

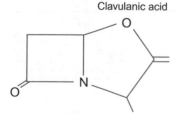

Clavulanic acid

Figure 8.8 Skeleton structure of *clavulanic acid.*

Side-effects of β-lactam antibacterials

Probably the most serious side-effect of the penicillins is allergic hypersensitivity. Up to 10% of the population is susceptible to adverse reactions from *penicillin* and its derivatives and can suffer from rashes and fever. In a few individuals, the reaction can be more severe, resulting in **anaphylaxis**, but this is fortunately quite rare. Individuals who already suffer from allergies, hay fever and asthma are at greater risk from hypersensitivity reactions.

> **Anaphylaxis** is a condition where a normally innocuous substance causes a severe immune response, resulting in general vasodilation and oedema in the lungs. This results in a fall in blood pressure and difficulty with breathing.

> **IN PRACTICE**
>
> Sometimes antibacterial drugs can be the causative agent of bacterial diseases. *Clostridium difficile* in the gut is relatively unaffected by many of the broad spectrum antibacterials that may kill other commensals thus allowing *C. difficile* to flourish, free from competition. The proliferation of *C. difficile* can cause inflammation of the gut and even septicaemia.

Antibacterials 2: drugs targeting ribosomes

There are many well-known antibacterial drugs in this category such as **tetracyclines**, **aminoglycosides**, *chloramphenicol* and *erythromycin*. All of these drugs target bacterial ribosomes and prevent the bacterium from producing proteins.

The process of protein synthesis was discussed briefly in Chapter 1. A section of DNA, called a gene, codes for a protein and when the cell wants to make a particular protein, the gene is copied from DNA into mRNA. This is transported from the nucleus into the cytoplasm of the cell where the ribosomes translate the mRNA into a protein. The code contained in the mRNA tells the ribosome the order of the amino acids that make up the protein. Figure 8.9 is a greatly simplified portrayal of the process. It shows the ribosome tracking along a length of mRNA and reading the code. Each small section of mRNA contains the code for one of the 20 amino acids. The ribosome reads the code and then selects a corresponding free amino acid from the cytoplasm and adds it to the growing chain of amino acids.

The process of protein synthesis is of vital importance to any organism and any drug that interferes with the process will cause major problems for that organism. Growth in particular will be inhibited because cells need to make new proteins in order for them to undergo cell division. This is why drugs that target ribosomes inhibit bacterial growth – in other words, they are bacteriostatic.

Drugs such as the tetracyclines, aminoglycosides, etc., are able to target bacterial ribosomes because they are slightly different from the ribosomes found in eukaryotic

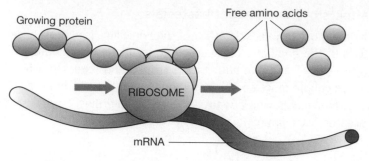

Figure 8.9 A ribosome translates the code contained in a section of mRNA and assembles a chain of amino acids that form a protein.

human cells. This difference in structure, although relatively small, is just enough difference to make a target for antibacterial drugs.

> ### KEY FACT
>
> Bacterial ribosomes are slightly different from human ribosomes and therefore make a target for antibacterial drugs.

Tetracyclines

This group includes *tetracycline* itself, *doxycycline*, *minocycline*, *oxytetracycline* and *tigecycline*. These are broad spectrum antibacterials that are useful against a variety of organisms that can cause various diseases such as urinary tract, respiratory and oral infections. They are also widely used for *Chlamydia* infections and against *Neisseria meningitidis*, the causative agent of bacterial meningitis.

Resistance to tetracyclines is becoming increasingly problematical as bacteria find new ways of overcoming the drug. Many bacteria are able to pump the drug out of their cells and some produce a protein that appears to shield the ribosome from the effects of tetracycline. Others produce an enzyme that modifies tetracyclines, rendering them ineffective.

> ### IN PRACTICE
>
> Tetracyclines act as **chelating** agents for calcium in the body. In other words, they bind to Ca^{2+} and prevent its use in physiological processes. They are contra-indicated in children under 12 and women who are pregnant or breast-feeding who need plenty of calcium, especially for bone growth.

Aminoglycosides

This group includes *gentamicin*, *amikacin*, *neomycin* and *tobramycin*. None of this group is absorbed well orally and they are generally delivered IV or by intramuscular (IM) injection. They are effective against Gram-positive and Gram-negative aerobic bacteria and used for serious systemic infections, including bacterial meningitis. All aminoglycosides can cause damage to the inner ear and also damage to the nephrons of the kidney, so care is cautioned in those with renal problems. *Streptomycin*, a related drug, is reserved for tuberculosis.

> **CASE STUDY**
>
> Recently discharged from hospital where she underwent a hip replacement, Pam complains of a fever and severe discomfort when urinating. You suspect a urinary tract infection, possibly involving *E. coli*, one of the most common causative agents. What might be a suitable treatment?

Comment on case study There is just a possibility that the UTI was acquired in hospital and therefore might be a resistant strain. However, antibacterials effective against resistant bacteria should be reserved for infections where resistance is established. *Co-amoxiclav* might be a suitable choice where resistance is only a possibility. Because *clavulanic acid* has no antibacterial action, bacteria cannot develop resistance against it.

Macrolides, lincosamides and chloramphenicol

Erythromycin is perhaps the most widely used of the macrolides and as it has a similar spectrum of activity to *penicillin*, it is a useful alternative for patients allergic to *penicillin*.

Clindamycin is the sole representative of the lincosamides, effective against Gram-positive cocci, it is recommended for staphylococcal joint and bone infections and peritonitis. *Chloramphenicol* is a potent broad spectrum drug that is reserved for serious systemic infections because it can severely suppress bone marrow activity in some individuals, resulting in anaemia. *Chloramphenicol* preparations are also available for topical application as eye and ear drops.

Antibacterials 3: fluoroquinolones

Sometimes abbreviated to **quinolones**, this broad spectrum group includes *ciprofloxacin, levofloxacin, moxifloxacin, norfloxacin* and *ofloxacin*. They work by inhibiting **topoisomerase II**, an enzyme involved in uncoiling the DNA helix during **replication** to make new DNA, or **transcription** to make mRNA. The fluoroquinolones therefore prevent both cell division and protein synthesis. The group is particularly active against Gram-negative organisms in the treatment of infections of the respiratory and urinary tracts. *Ciprofloxacin* is used in the treatment of some sexually transmitted infections such as gonorrhoea and chlamydia.

> **Replication** of DNA is the production of new DNA during cell (in this case, bacterial) division. **Transcription** is the copying of a section of DNA into mRNA during protein synthesis.

Antibacterials 4: other antibacterial drugs

There are many different types of antibacterial drugs listed in the *British National Formulary*, some of which are used regularly for common problems while others are for rarer diseases or have highly specific indications. It would be quite easy to devote a whole book to antimicrobial drugs, but as we have only one chapter, we will have to be selective and conclude this section on antibacterials with a brief summary of those drugs that are most regularly encountered in clinical practice.

Vancomycin and *teicoplanin* are used in the treatment of endocarditis and other serious infections from Gram-positive bacteria. These drugs inhibit peptidoglycan synthesis, causing rupture of the bacterial cell wall, but by a different mechanism from the β-lactam antibacterials.

Trimethoprim is used for urinary tract and lung infections. It works by inhibiting an enzyme responsible for synthesising DNA which prevents bacterial replication.

Rifampicin is useful for endocarditis and other serious infections, including tuberculosis and legionnaire's disease. It inhibits an enzyme that transcribes DNA into mRNA and so halts protein synthesis. *Rifampicin* is a potent inducer of hepatic enzymes that can break down other drugs, including oral contraceptives, lowering their serum concentration.

Metronidazole is used against anaerobic bacterial infections, including *Helicobacter pylori*. Its mechanism of action is not fully understood but it probably disrupts DNA and inhibits DNA replication.

Nitrofurantoin treats urinary tract infections. Its mechanism of action is not fully understood.

A QUICK RECAP on antibacterial drugs

- Antibacterial drugs target structures that are different from human cells in bacteria.
- Some antibacterials are broad spectrum and target a wide range of bacteria. Some are narrow spectrum, targeting specific groups.
- Beta-lactam antibacterials include the penicillins, cephalosporins and carbapenems.
- Beta-lactam drugs block an enzyme involved in the production of peptidoglycan, an essential component of the bacterial cell wall. This bactericidal action causes the cell wall to rupture.
- Bacterial resistance is often due to bacteria-producing enzymes such as β-lactamases that denature the β-lactam ring of β-lactam drugs.
- Tetracyclines, aminoglycosides and related drugs target bacterial ribosomes and inhibit protein synthesis. This bacteriostatic action prevents replication.
- Fluoroquinolones prevent both cell division and protein synthesis.
- Many other antibacterial drugs are available, each having its own mechanism of action against the bacteria it targets.

Fungi

Fungi are a diverse group of organisms and the majority are non-pathogenic – some, such as chanterelles, are quite tasty and nice to eat. Other fungi, such as the yeast *Saccharomyces cerevisiae*, are used in brewing wines and beers and baking bread. Those that are pathogenic tend to be at the small end of the fungal size spectrum, often, as with *Candida albicans*, single-celled yeasts. Common pathogenic fungi include:

- *Candida albicans* – thrush (vaginal and oral)
- *Trichophyton* – athlete's foot
- *Aspergillus* – aspergillosis
- *Tinea capitis* – ringworm of the scalp and hair
- *Tinea corporis, T. cruris and T. pedis* – skin and nail infections
- *Cryptococcus neoformans* – cryptococcosis

Fungal infections in healthy individuals generally tend to be topical in nature and not life-threatening. **Ringworm**, thrush and **athlete's foot** are common and relatively easily treated, responding to antifungal drugs discussed below. The main danger from fungal infections is with those who are already severely ill or immunocompromised. Here fungi act as opportunistic pathogens and can cause serious and life-threatening conditions. *Candida albicans* is an example of an organism that rarely causes severe problems in healthy individuals beyond occasional vulvovaginal **candidiasis** (thrush) in females. However, **systemic candidiasis** can develop in those whose immune system has been suppressed such as **human immunodeficiency virus** (HIV) infected patients with **acquired immuno-deficiency syndrome** (AIDS) or cancer patients receiving immunosuppressant drugs. This is a very serious disease with a high mortality rate that can result in organs of the body becoming infected. Systemic candidiasis is generally not encountered outside the intensive care unit.

Fungi are eukaryotic organisms, which means that their cell structure is similar to our own, and this makes them difficult to target with drugs. Certainly, antibacterial drugs have no effect on them because bacterial targets are not found in fungi. However, as with bacteria, an antifungal drug has to target fungal structures that are different from those found in human cells.

Amphotericin and *nystatin*

A key fungal target is the fungal cell membranes which contain **ergosterol** rather than the cholesterol found in human membranes. Like cholesterol, ergosterol is essential for the stability of the cell membrane. The antifungal drugs *amphotericin* and *nystatin* have an affinity for ergosterol, and in binding to it they disrupt the integrity of the membrane, causing the cell to lyse and die. *Amphotericin* is used for severe systemic fungal infections such as systemic candidiasis and cryptococcosis.

It is acknowledged to be quite toxic and must be used with care. *Nystatin* is used for intestinal, vaginal and skin fungal infections.

Flucytosine is another antifungal drug that is used for serious systemic infections. It inhibits the fungal enzyme **thymidylate synthetase** that has a role in protein synthesis.

Fluconazole and *miconazole* (azoles) target fungal enzymes responsible for the synthesis of ergosterol. Membranes lose their integrity and this inhibits replication. *Fluconazole* is used for a wide range of fungal infections, topical and systemic including oral and vaginal candidiasis. *Miconazole* is used for topical mouth and skin infections.

Griseofulvin acts against fungal microtubules and prevents cell division. It is used for skin, scalp and nail infections.

Caspofungin is a relatively recent drug, used in the treatment of serious systemic fungal infections such as **aspergillosis**. It inhibits the synthesis of a fungal poly-saccharide, an essential component of the cell wall.

Unwanted effects of antifungals are usually mild and can include the general side-effect of nausea, vomiting, diarrhoea and rashes. Some of the azoles are cautioned in patients with hepatic impairment and congestive heart failure (see BNF). Parenteral amphotericin also has many cautions (see BNF).

CASE STUDY

Darren is an IV drug user who has recently been diagnosed with HIV infection. He presents at surgery with white plaques on his tongue and gums. You suspect oral candidiasis. What would you prescribe?

Comment on case study *Fluconazole* is the drug of choice here and should resolve the problem. If Darren is susceptible to fungal infections, vigilance will be necessary as the HIV infection progresses because candidiasis and cryptococcosis can become invasive, causing serious problems in immunocompromised patients.

8.4　Viruses

Viruses are very, very small – around 10-100 nm (1000 nm = 1 µm) so they can only be viewed with an electron microscope. They are **obligate cellular parasites**, meaning that they can only reproduce after invading a host cell and they are invariably pathogenic to their hosts. Most organisms are susceptible to attack by viruses; animals, plants, fungi and even bacteria are all viral targets. Viruses tend to be very specific to their hosts so, for example, humans cannot contract cat flu from their pets or hydrangea mosaic virus from their pot plants.

Common pathogenic viruses include:

- **Rhinovirus** – common cold
- **Orthomyxovirus** – influenza
- **Paramyxovirus** – measles
- **Varicella-zoster** – chickenpox and shingles (neural varicella-zoster)
- **Norovirus** – gastroenteritis
- **Rotavirus** – diarrhoea (especially in children)
- **Astrovirus** – gastroenteritis
- **Papillomavirus** – genital warts
- **Coronavirus** – Severe Acute Respiratory Syndrome (SARS)
- **Human immunodeficiency virus** – HIV – AIDS

DID YOU KNOW . . . that viruses are so remote from other kingdoms and their relationships so problematical that they do not take normal nomenclature as devised by Carl Linnaeus (1707–1778)? These binomial (double) names identify organisms by their genus and species name, respectively, as in *Homo sapiens* and *Escherichia coli*.

Viruses are very simple in their structure – often just a strand of DNA or RNA in a protein capsule or lipid envelope. Figure 8.10 shows a typical structure of an encapsulated virus but note that they exhibit great structural diversity.

Because viruses reproduce inside host cells, they are difficult to attack with drugs. A few drugs have been developed which target some of the proteins unique to viruses but our main defence is **vaccination** which preprogrammes the body's immune system to defend it against a particular virus. A few drugs are available for the treatment of **influenza** and **respiratory syncytial virus** infections, generally for use only in high-risk patients.

Infection with human immunodeficiency virus (HIV) produces a complex, incurable disease that results in a weakening of the body's immune response, with the eventual onset of a suite of diseases common in immunocompromised patients

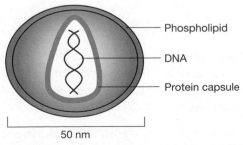

Figure 8.10 Typical structure of an encapsulated virus.

known as acquired immunodeficiency syndrome, or AIDS. This disease has spread inexorably across the world, infecting millions of people, especially in developing countries where sexual education is inadequate or ineffective. The development of drugs to combat HIV has been steady and while none of them produces a cure, it is now possible to slow the progression of HIV infection and give infected individuals a reasonable quality of life. It is an indication of the effort put into developing a cure for HIV that there are more drugs available to treat HIV than there are for all other viral infections combined. Generally anti-HIV drugs target viral enzymes or processes associated with viral replication in the cell. The drugs are always given in combinations termed **HAART** (highly active antiretroviral treatment). As management of HIV is a specialist clinical area, it would not be appropriate to discuss it in more detail here.

Herpesvirus infections

These infections are caused by viruses of the herpes group. Herpes simplex causes cold sores, conjunctivitis, mouth ulcers and genital infections. Varicella-zoster virus causes shingles and chicken pox. Drugs used to treat herpes infections are of the *aciclovir* (acyclovir) family that inhibit **viral RNA polymerase**, an enzyme that produces viral proteins. Protein synthesis is halted and so is viral replication.

CASE STUDY

Charlie arrives in surgery with a streaming head cold. He says he feels 'rough' and wants some antibiotics to make him feel better and get him back to work. What would you do?

Comment on case study Charlie's problem is caused by a virus and is not bacterial in origin. The word *antibiotic* is popularly used to refer to antibacterial drugs and these will have no effect on Charlie's viral infection – in fact, there are currently no drugs available to treat the common cold. Having satisfied yourself that the problem is indeed a cold and that Charlie is not vulnerable to complications, he should be advised to stay at home, keep warm and not return to work until the symptoms have gone.

8.5   Protozoa

This group of single-celled organisms cause some unpleasant diseases that include malaria, amoebiasis and leishmaniasis. Fortunately, most of these diseases are usually found in the tropics so are less likely to be encountered outside a clinical setting specialising in tropical diseases.

- Trichomoniasis is a fairly common sexually transmitted disease caused by the organism *Trichomonas vaginalis*. Treatment is by **metronidazole** or **tinidazole**.

- Toxoplasmosis is a disease caused by the protozoan *Toxoplasma gondii*. It is generally a self-limiting disease that can be caught from domestic pets. Pregnant women and immunocompromised patients are at more risk and require specialist clinical expertise.

8.6   Helminths (worms)

The **threadworm** (*Enterobius vermicularis*) is probably the most common cause of **helmintic** disease in the UK. The worms go through a cycle that requires the re-ingestion of worm eggs that are laid around the area of the anus. **Pruritus** (itching) results in scratching and the eggs can be transferred under the fingernails to the mouth – thus repeating the cycle. The obvious treatment involves strict hygiene followed by a dose of *mebendazole* or *piperazine*.

Mebendazole inhibits glucose uptake in the worms and *piperazine* paralyses muscles in the worms, allowing them to be expelled alive.

A QUICK RECAP on drugs for fungal, viral, protozoan and helmintic infections

- Antifungal drugs mainly target the fungal cell membrane that contains ergosterol rather than the cholesterol found in human cells.

- Viruses are obligate cellular parasites and therefore difficult to target with drugs. Vaccination is the most effective way to prevent viral infection.

- There are relatively few antiviral drugs for common viral infections such as colds and flu. Many drugs have been developed to combat HIV.

- Trichomoniasis, a sexually transmitted disease, is the most common protozoan infection in the UK, along with toxoplasmosis, a disease transmitted from domestic animals such as cats.

- Threadworms are relatively common in the UK, especially in children. They can be eliminated with good hygiene and drugs such as *mebendazole* or *piperazine*.

RUNNING WORDS

Here are some of the technical terms that were included in this chapter. Read through them one by one and tick them off when you are sure that you understand them.

Acquired immunodeficiency syndrome (AIDS) p. 199
Aerobes p. 189
Aminoglycosides p. 195
Anaerobes p. 189
Anaphylaxis p. 195
Antimicrobial p. 183
Aspergillosis p. 200
Astrovirus p. 201
Athlete's foot p. 199
Azoles p. 200
Bacilli p. 189
Bacterial p. 182
Bacterial resistance p. 193
Bactericidal p. 191
Bacteriostatic p. 191
β-lactam p. 191
β-lactamases p. 192
β-lactam ring p. 192
Blind therapy p. 191
Broad spectrum p. 191
Candidiasis p. 182
Carbapenems p. 192
Cephalosporinases p. 188
Cephalosporins p. 188
Chelating p. 196
Christian Gram p. 188
Cocci p. 189
Commensals p. 187
Coronavirus p. 201

Crystal violet p. 188
Diplococci p. 189
Endocarditis p. 191
Endospores p. 186
Ergosterol p. 199
Eukaryotes p. 185
Facultative anaerobes p. 189
Flagella p. 186
Fimbriae p. 186
Fungal p. 182
Gram negative p. 188
Gram positive p. 188
HAART p. 202
Helminths p. 183
Helmintic p. 203
Human immunodeficiency virus p. 199
Influenza p. 201
Lyse p. 192
Meningitis p. 191
Microbes p. 182
Microorganisms helminths p. 183
Motile p. 186
Narrow spectrum p. 191
Norovirus p. 201
Obligate p. 186
Obligate cellular parasites p. 200
Opportunist pathogens p. 187
Orthomyxovirus p. 201

Papillomavirus p. 201
Paramyxovirus p. 201
Penicillinases p. 188
Penicillins p. 188
Peptidoglycan p. 188
Prokaryotes p. 185
Protoctista p. 184
Pruritus p. 203
Quinolones p. 197
Replication p. 197
Respiratory syncytial virus p. 201
Rhinovirus p. 182
Ringworm p. 199
Rotavirus p. 201
Selective toxicity p. 191
Septicaemia p. 191
Staphylococci p. 189
Streptococci p. 189
Systemic candidiasis p. 199
Tetracyclines p. 195
Threadworm p. 203
Thrush p. 182
Thymidylate synthetase p. 200
Topoisomerase II p. 197
Transcription p. 197
Transpeptidase p. 188
Vaccination p. 201
Varicella-zoster p. 201
Viral p. 182
Viral RNA polymerase p. 202

REFERENCES AND FURTHER RECOMMENDED READING

All recommended websites are open access (but free registration is sometimes required).

NICE guidelines on infection control – http://www.nice.org.uk/Guidance/CG2

National Electronic Library of Infection – http://www.neli.org.uk/

NHS Website (search for specific infection) – http://www.nhs.uk/Conditions/

Your turn to try

Now you have finished reading through this chapter try answering these questions to see how much you have learned.

The answers to these questions are at the end of the book on page 286.

1 Name the four groups of microbes that can cause microbial infection.

2 Which was the first group of microbes to evolve on earth?

3 What do you understand by the terms 'prokaryote' and 'eukaryote'?

4 Name three factors by which we can classify bacteria.

5 What is the name of the structural glycoprotein found in bacterial cell walls?

6 How do penicillins and cephalosporins kill bacteria?

7 What is the chief way that bacteria become resistant to penicillins and cephalosporins?

8 How does clavulanic acid help to evade bacterial resistance?

9 What is the difference between a bactericidal and a bacteriostatic drug?

10 What bacterial structure do tetracyclines and aminoglycosides target?

11 Why are tetracyclines contra-indicated in pregnant women?

12 What is the main target for antifungal drugs?

13 Why are viruses so difficult to target with drugs?

14 What is the most effective way to prevent viral infection?

15 What drug can treat both protozoan and bacterial infection?

Answers to questions on page 184

1 A fungus (single-celled yeast).
2 Meticillin resistant *Staphylococcus aureus*.
3 A bacterium.
4 A virus.
5 No – a cold is caused by a virus and penicillin is only effective against bacteria.

Chapter 9

Disorders and drugs of the respiratory system

AIMS

By the time you have finished the chapter you should be able to understand:

1 The **physiology** – the structure and function of the respiratory system.
2 The **pathology** – those disorders and pathologies associated with the respiratory system.
3 The **pharmacology** – the action of the major drug groups used in the treatment of respiratory disorders and pathologies.

CONTENTS

The chapter contains some brief case studies and finishes off with self-test questions to ensure that you have understood the physiology of the respiratory system, associated disorders and the pharmacology of drugs used to treat those disorders.

IN PRACTICE

Whatever your branch of clinical practice, you will encounter patients with respiratory problems. **Asthma** is a common disease that generally originates in childhood and often persists into later life. **Cystic fibrosis** is an incurable genetic disease that can affect the lungs. It is less common than asthma but is also one that can continue from childhood into adulthood. **Bronchitis** and **emphysema** are relatively common chronic respiratory diseases that predominantly affect older people. All of the diseases just mentioned tend to be chronic problems that can persist for years but there are also many respiratory problems of a shorter duration. Some, such as **pneumonia** can be very serious, especially in the elderly. Other diseases are unpleasant but usually less serious and most people at some time will have succumbed to a cough or chest infection. Because the lungs are so important to the normal physiological functioning of the individual, any disease that interferes with gas exchange in the lungs can have a profound effect on the rest of the body. It is important, therefore, that you understand the basic physiology of the lungs, how associated pathologies can cause problems, and how the drugs at our disposal can help patients with respiratory problems.

Introduction

We all need to breathe regularly, between 12 and 15 times a minute from the moment we are born until the final moment of our lives – often referred to as 'our last breath'. Breathing delivers fresh oxygen-containing air into the lungs and removes carbon dioxide. If we stop breathing for any reason the consequences are extremely serious indeed because, after a few minutes, we die – and things don't get more serious than that! Healthy lungs are very important indeed to the well-being of the individual and any disease that compromises the efficient functioning of the lungs is going to cause problems. The incidence of lung diseases in the UK has changed over the past decades, reflecting changes in wealth, health and lifestyle. **Chronic obstructive pulmonary diseases** (COPD), such as bronchitis and emphysema, were originally industrial in origin, caused by poor working conditions in polluted factories. These days, there are fewer factories in the UK and Health and Safety regulations are much more tightly controlled. Even so, we have over 500,000 people in the UK with COPD. Chronic bronchitis and emphysema are still with us, but cigarette smoking is now the prime cause. With a cleaner, less-polluted environment it might be thought that lung disease generally would steadily be reducing in incidence but no, because for one disease, asthma, the incidence is steadily increasing. Fifty years ago, asthma was relatively uncommon, but today the NHS website tells us that around five million people are being treated for asthma in the UK.

In this chapter we will first look at the anatomy and physiology of the respiratory system and then examine some common diseases such as asthma, bronchitis and cough. Finally we look at the drugs available to restore normal function when problems occur. There are also some diseases of the respiratory system that are caused by bacterial infections, such as pneumonia as well as viral infections, such as severe acute respiratory syndrome (SARS) and influenza. These require specialist treatment beyond the scope of this introductory book but some of the antimicrobial drugs used to treat these infections were covered in Chapter 8. Lung cancer is another all too common disease, generally caused by cigarette smoking. As with lung infections, treatment requires the use of specialist drugs which will be covered in more advanced pharmacology books.

WHERE ARE WE STARTING FROM?

In this chapter we will examine the respiratory system and the drugs that treat common disorders such as asthma, bronchitis and emphysema. Hopefully, you already understand the basic anatomy and physiology of the respiratory system but let's start off with the usual short quiz to find out how much you do know before we begin:

1 What is the name of the main airway that connects the mouth to the lungs?

_____

2 Do we extract oxygen or carbon dioxide from the air we breathe in?

_____

3 When the ribs rise and the diaphragm falls, does air enter or leave the lungs?

_____

4 What is the name of the small air sacs at the end of the bronchioles where gas exchange takes place?

_____

5 What is the name of the membranes that surround the lungs?

_____

Answers are at the end of the chapter on page 225.

How did you do? We cover the basics of the respiratory system at the beginning of this chapter but if you really struggled with these questions then it might be an idea to refresh your knowledge from your physiology book.

9.1 The anatomy and physiology of the respiratory system

The function of the respiratory system is primarily to facilitate the transfer of gas between the body and the atmosphere. As we have seen in previous chapters, oxygen is a gas that is required by every cell of the body to make energy in the form of ATP. Without oxygen, cells are unable to make ATP in sufficient quantities and if the supply of oxygen is cut off for long enough then cells will die. This is what happens in heart attacks when a blood clot in the coronary arteries deprives heart muscle of oxygen-carrying blood and cells start dying (unless the paramedics arrive quickly with thrombolytic drugs). The removal of carbon dioxide is an equally important task of the lungs. Carbon dioxide produced during cellular respiration is carried by the blood from the tissues to the lungs where it is disposed of into the atmosphere. It will thus be obvious that any problem with the lungs will quickly affect gas exchange and, consequently, gas levels in the body. A fall in oxygen or a rise in carbon dioxide levels are both potentially serious and compensatory mechanisms exist in the body to restore normal gas levels. However, these mechanisms are dependent on lungs that are functioning normally.

The structure of the respiratory system facilitates the movement of air between the outside of the body and the **alveoli** of the lungs where **gas exchange** takes place. Figure 9.1 shows the gross structure of the respiratory system.

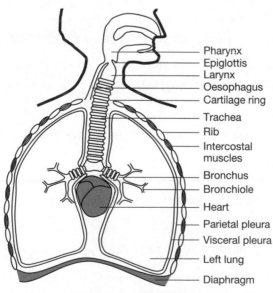

Pharynx
Epiglottis
Larynx
Oesophagus
Cartilage ring

Trachea
Rib
Intercostal muscles

Bronchus
Bronchiole

Heart

Parietal pleura
Visceral pleura

Left lung

Diaphragm

Figure 9.1 The structure of the respiratory system. Note that many branches of the bronchioles have been omitted for clarity, as have some of the ribs.

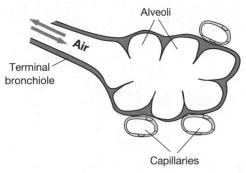

Figure 9.2 Alveoli and associated capillaries form the respiratory membrane.

After entering the mouth or nose, air moves down the trachea to a point just underneath the midpoint of the sternum, where the trachea branches into the left and right **bronchi**. Each **bronchus** then divides and subdivides into **bronchioles** and these continue to divide, around 20 or so times, getting smaller with each division. At the end of the smallest bronchioles are the alveoli, small air sacs where gas exchange takes place. There are millions of alveoli in each lung, each surrounded by a network of small blood vessels called capillaries (Figure 9.2). The walls of the alveoli are only one cell thick, as are the adjacent capillaries, which means that air and blood are brought into very close proximity, separated by less than 1.0 μm. This area is called the **respiratory membrane**.

DID YOU KNOW . . . that the adult human lungs contain almost 500 million alveoli, giving an average area of around 80 m² - about half the size of a tennis court? This large area provides spare capacity when there needs to be a dramatic increase in gas exchange - for example, during vigorous exercise.

Gas exchange in the alveoli

Gas exchange takes place across the very thin respiratory membrane formed by the cells of the alveoli and capillaries. In the alveoli, the concentration of oxygen is high because breathing has brought in fresh air from the atmosphere. In the pulmonary capillaries, the concentration of oxygen in the blood is low because the tissue cells have extracted much of the oxygen to make energy in the form of ATP. This means that there is a **diffusion gradient** between the alveoli and the blood in the capillaries. Oxygen will therefore diffuse down this gradient from the alveoli to the blood (Figure 9.3).

The blood in the pulmonary capillaries has a high concentration of carbon dioxide because the cells of the tissues have produced carbon dioxide to make energy. In the alveoli, the concentration is low because breathing has brought in fresh air from the atmosphere and this contains very little carbon dioxide. This means that there is a diffusion gradient between the alveoli and the blood in

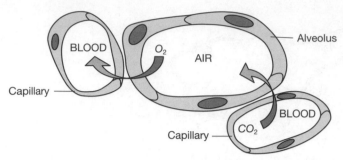

Figure 9.3 The diffusion of oxygen and carbon dioxide across the respiratory membrane.

the capillaries. Carbon dioxide will therefore diffuse down this gradient from the blood to the alveoli (Figure 9.3).

Diffusion gradient is the difference in concentration of a substance such as a gas or an ion, separated by a permeable membrane. The substance tends to diffuse across the membrane from the area of high concentration to the area of low concentration – until the concentrations on either side of the membrane are equal.

Ventilation and compliance

Inspiration is the movement of air into the lungs and requires the contraction of the **external intercostal** muscles that cause the ribs to rise and the flattening of the **diaphragm**. These two actions increase the volume of the lungs while, at the same time, decreasing the pressure. Air flows into the lungs down a pressure gradient from the higher atmospheric pressure outside to the lower pressure in the lungs.

    Expiration is the movement of air out of the lungs and this also involves changes in volumes and pressures. However, in breathing when the body is at rest, no muscular effort or energy is required to contract the lungs because, being elastic in nature, they recoil automatically from their expanded state.

ANOTHER WAY TO PICTURE THIS

Think of a bath sponge, which is actually quite similar in structure to the lungs. If you stretch the sponge, as in inspiration, it will recoil of its own accord when released. The 'stretchability' of the lungs is called **compliance**.

The **internal intercostal** muscles, while not being used in quiet breathing, are necessary for forced expiration such as when coughing or during heavy exercise.

    Healthy lungs with good compliance recoil automatically and easily, but certain disease conditions such as emphysema, bronchitis, tuberculosis and cystic fibrosis can compromise this process. **Mucus** that is produced in diseases such as bronchitis and asthma can partially block airways and result in ventilation problems.

Mucus is a viscous, slippery liquid that lines the mucous membranes of the body such as those of the respiratory, digestive and reproductive systems. Note the difference in spelling between the substance 'mucus' and the 'mucous' membranes that secrete it.

Respiratory defences and maintenance

In the airways of the lungs, a mechanism exists for removing the bacteria, dust and detritus that we inevitably breathe in each day. Goblet cells in the walls of the bronchioles produce the thin layer of mucus that lines the trachea, bronchi and bronchioles. This mucus is constantly moved along by tiny cilia, hair-like projections on the epithelial cells that line the respiratory tract. This mucus traps any foreign matter that has entered the lungs and transports it to the top of the trachea where it is usually swallowed (Figure 9.4).

In the alveoli, white blood cells called alveolar macrophages patrol the alveoli and destroy any bacteria that they find.

The control of breathing and compensatory mechanisms

When we are going about our daily tasks we are rarely conscious of the fact that we are breathing in and out around 15 times each minute. Sometimes, when we are at the gym or running for a bus we might notice that we are 'out of breath' and breathing more heavily and more rapidly than normally. These are examples of the control and compensatory mechanisms that maintain breathing and ensure adequate and efficient gas exchange in the alveoli of the lungs.

The maintenance of normal, regular breathing is via the respiratory centres of the brain stem. These set a steady rhythm that maintains the rhythmical breathing in the lungs via efferent nerves that control the intercostal muscles and diaphragm. As these muscles steadily contract and relax, air is moved in and out of the lungs, bringing in oxygen and removing carbon dioxide. When we exercise, however, we need more oxygen for the muscles to make their ATP and in the process we

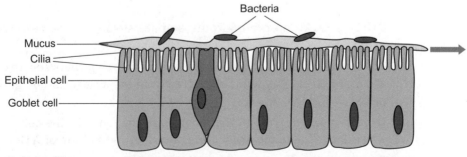

Figure 9.4 Cilia on epithelial cells remove bacteria trapped in mucus from the respiratory tract.

produce more carbon dioxide that must be disposed of into the atmosphere. The rate and depth of breathing is increased to facilitate this need for increased gas exchange. The trigger for this change in rate is, perhaps surprisingly, the increase in blood carbon dioxide levels rather than a fall in oxygen. This increase is detected by **chemoreceptors** in the medulla of the brain stem, which stimulates the rate and depth of breathing to pull more oxygen into the body and get rid of more carbon dioxide. When we stop exercising, levels of carbon dioxide fall and the rate and depth of breathing returns to normal.

KEY FACT

The carbon dioxide level in the blood is the main driver of breathing. Exercise causes CO_2 levels to rise and this causes an increase in the rate and depth of breathing.

In **chronic obstructive pulmonary disease** (COPD), such as **bronchitis** and **emphysema**, a condition can develop where the patient's breathing is being maintained by what is called '**hypoxic drive**'. COPD is a long-term condition where gas exchange is continuously compromised, resulting sometimes in chronically high levels of carbon dioxide in the blood. Eventually the respiratory centres may start to disregard CO_2 as a stimulus for breathing and instead rely on low levels of oxygen as the prime driver of respiration.

IN PRACTICE

When on hypoxic drive, the breathing of a COPD patient is being maintained by low levels of oxygen. This means it can be dangerous to suddenly give supplementary oxygen because the sudden rise in blood oxygen levels can remove the stimulus to breathe, resulting in respiratory failure.

Chemoreceptors are special receptor organs at the terminals of afferent neurons that detect changes in the chemical composition of the surrounding environment.

A QUICK RECAP on the anatomy and physiology of the respiratory system

- The prime function of the lungs is gas exchange between the body and atmospheric air. Oxygen is extracted from the air and carbon dioxide is disposed of into the air.

- Oxygen is transported in the blood from the lungs to the cells of the body where it is used in the production of energy in the form of ATP.

- Carbon dioxide is produced by cells when they make ATP and is transported in the blood to the lungs where it is disposed of into the atmosphere.

- At the end of the terminal bronchioles are small air sacs called alveoli that form the respiratory membrane. This is where gas exchange between the air and the blood takes place.
- Breathing in and out is by movement of the ribs and diaphragm which, together, create pressure gradients that facilitate the movement of air.
- The lungs are kept clean by the production of mucus that traps bacteria and detritus from the air. The mucus is steadily moved out of the lungs by the ciliated epithelial cells that line the respiratory tract.
- The prime driver of breathing is the level of CO_2 in the blood. As levels rise so the rate and depth of breathing increases to remove CO_2 from the body – and bring in more O_2.

9.2 Disorders of the respiratory system

Asthma

Asthma is an inflammatory disease characterised by hypersensitivity of the airways resulting in periodic **bronchospasm** (narrowing of the airways). It is one of the most common respiratory diseases in the UK, where it affects around five million people, many of them children. The incidence of asthma has increased steadily over the past decades, which may be surprising considering that the atmosphere in the UK is now less polluted and health care has improved. The reason for this increase is not fully understood but is believed to be linked to the fact that our immune system is now challenged less often in infancy by disease-causing pathogens. Vaccination has all but eliminated many diseases such as **diphtheria**, **measles** and **polio** that were once common and our homes are generally clean and centrally heated. Consequently, children now are just not exposed to the immunological challenges of previous generations and somehow this may result in the immune system becoming more sensitive to challenges from substances such as dust mites and animal fur that present no real threat to their health. Whatever the reason, asthma is a very common disease and many drugs have been developed to make the lives of those who suffer from the problem more bearable.

In asthma, the bronchi and bronchioles become inflamed and sensitive to **allergens** such as dust mites, animal fur, pollen and a variety of otherwise innocuous substances. In addition to allergens, environmental factors such as cold air, stress and exercise can also exacerbate the problems of the asthma sufferer. When the asthmatic is exposed to particular allergens, this can cause an **asthma attack**. The allergen is carried into the airways where it is recognised by mast cells of the immune system in the epithelium of the bronchioles. There then follows a sequence of events, typical of the inflammatory response that we examined in Chapter 6. Mast cells release chemical mediators such as histamine,

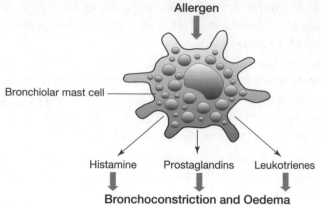

Figure 9.5 Stimulation of a mast cell in the bronchioles by allergen causes the release of histamine, prostaglandins and leukotrienes, resulting in bronchoconstriction and oedema.

prostaglandins and leukotrienes (Figure 9.5). This results in bronchoconstriction caused by contraction of the smooth muscle that surrounds the bronchioles. Plasma leaks out of the small blood vessels causing oedema and goblet cells in the bronchiole epithelium to release copious amounts of mucus. All of this has the effect of narrowing the airways and stimulating nerve endings, resulting in the feeling of irritation. In addition to bronchoconstriction and oedema, leukotrienes have a role in the attraction of **eosinophils**, white blood cells that amplify the inflammatory response and may eventually cause damage to the epithelial lining of the bronchioles.

> **Allergens** are substances that trigger allergic reactions. The immune system recognises and responds to allergens by releasing chemical mediators such as histamine that are responsible for the symptoms of an allergic response such as swelling, sneezing and itching.

The onset of an asthma attack brings on **dyspnoea** (shortness of breath), tightness in the chest, coughing and wheezing – although symptoms will vary between individuals. Bronchoconstriction, swelling and excess mucus in the bronchioles impede the flow of air in and out of the lungs and this interferes with normal gas exchange in the alveoli. The uptake of oxygen into the blood is adversely affected as is the removal of carbon dioxide, levels of which are elevated, resulting in an urgency to increase the rate of ventilation. Unfortunately, this is hampered by the narrow airways, resulting in the shortness of breath and distress experienced during an asthma attack. The initial attack is often followed by a **late-phase response** several hours later. This also involves bronchoconstriction and an increase in airway sensitivity but the mechanism behind it is less well understood.

IN PRACTICE

Narrowed airways cause breathing difficulties and perhaps the easiest way to monitor the efficiency of a patient's lungs is with a **peak flow meter**, a small hand-held device into which the patient blows hard. A scale gives the rate at which air is being exhaled in litres per minute. The reading can be checked against standardised figures for the patient's sex, age and height.

Chronic obstructive pulmonary disease

Chronic obstructive pulmonary disease (COPD) includes bronchitis and emphysema and is characterised by a restriction of airflow both into and out of the lungs which develops over a period of time, perhaps months or years. COPD differs primarily from asthma in that the restriction is permanent rather than episodic and reversible as in asthma. Although the pathologies of bronchitis and emphysema are somewhat different, they have a common set of breathing-related symptoms, including . . .

- Chronic cough
- **Expectoration** (coughing-up) of mucus
- Breathlessness upon exertion
- Progressive reduction in the ability to exhale
- Increase in susceptibility to chest infections.

The main cause of both bronchitis and emphysema is many years of smoking and it is the toxic chemicals in the smoke that cause permanent damage to the lungs. In bronchitis, smoking triggers chronic inflammation that results in damage to the airways. The cilia, hair-like projections that move bacteria and foreign particles out of the lungs are damaged so that the lungs retain mucus. The mucous glands themselves become enlarged, resulting in an overproduction of mucus. Bacteria such as *Streptococcus pneumoniae*, *Haemophilus influenzae* and *Moraxella catarrhalis* become trapped in the excess mucus that accumulates in the lungs and this can result in chest infections. To add to the problem, **hypertrophy**, an overgrowth of the smooth muscle cells that surround the airways, will further restrict airflow. Figure 9.6 shows how oedema, mucus and hypertrophy can reduce the size of the bronchiolar **lumen** (air space).

In emphysema, the walls of the alveoli break down and this reduces the surface area of the respiratory membrane. Gas exchange is compromised, resulting in a lower intake of oxygen and a reduced removal of carbon dioxide. Bronchitis is a common complication of emphysema

Lumen is a term used to refer to the space enclosed by any of the hollow organs of the body such as the bronchioles, small intestine or blood vessels.

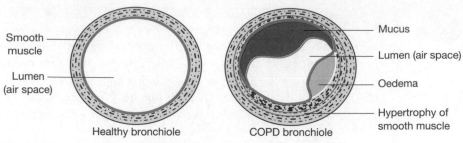

Figure 9.6 Mucus, oedema and hypertrophy of smooth muscle can combine to reduce the size of the bronchiolar lumen.

CASE STUDY

Jim is 55 and presents at the clinic with a cough that has been troubling him for weeks and he says that he is producing a lot of phlegm. His breathing is noisy and he complains that it gets worse when he climbs the stairs. He says he has given up smoking but his nicotine-stained fingers tell another story. What would you advise?

Comment on case study Jim's symptoms are indicative of early COPD. A peak flow test will give some indication of the state of his lungs. Jim needs to be honest about his smoking and perhaps be referred to a smoking-cessation clinic. If he can stop smoking now, there is a chance that the disease can be halted and he may be able to resume participation in normal physical activities.

Cough

The cough is a defensive mechanism that can expel foreign bodies and mucus from the airways. It can also be triggered by irritation of the airways due to inflammation and infection. Irritation usually results in a **dry cough** where no mucus is expelled whereas in infection, the cough more often produces mucus. Some drugs such as ACE inhibitors (as discussed in Chapter 5) can irritate the bronchioles, resulting in a dry cough. The cough mechanism itself is not well understood but is thought to operate via a poorly defined 'cough centre' in the brainstem. When this is activated, efferent nerves to the intercostal muscles of the ribs cause the rapid, forced expulsion of air, resulting in the familiar coughing sound.

A QUICK RECAP on disorders of the respiratory system

- **Asthma** is an inflammatory disease with hypersensitivity of the airways resulting in periodic **bronchospasm.**
- Symptoms of asthma are dyspnoea, coughing and wheezing and the production of excess mucus.
- The pathology of asthma involves the production of histamine, prostaglandins and leukotrienes that cause bronchoconstriction and oedema.

- Chronic obstructive pulmonary disease (COPD) includes bronchitis and emphysema, chronic diseases that affect the movement of air in and out of the lungs.
- In bronchitis, excess mucus and trapped bacteria lead to recurrent infections
- In emphysema there is an irreversible breakdown of the respiratory membrane in the alveoli resulting in impaired gas exchange. Oxygen levels in the blood fall and carbon dioxide levels rise.
- Cough is a natural defence mechanism that expels foreign bodies from the airways but is also triggered by infection and inflammation.

9.3 Drugs used in the management of respiratory system disorders

There are various types of drugs used in the treatment of respiratory disorders. Improving the movement of air through the bronchioles can be achieved by bronchodilators that relax the smooth muscle surrounding the bronchioles and both long and short-acting bronchodilators are available. Another approach is to reduce inflammation in the bronchioles which can help make the airways less sensitive as well as reducing oedema and mucus production. For those with chronic asthma, the BNF provides a recommended protocol that outlines the best choice and combination of drugs to ensure effective management of the disease. Acute, severe asthma attacks can be life threatening if the patient is unable to breathe properly and supplemental oxygen often needs to be administered as well as the specific bronchodilators discussed below.

Drug group 1: bronchodilators (indicated for asthma and COPD)

Bronchodilators 1: selective beta$_2$ agonists

These include *salbutamol, terbutaline, bambuterol, formoterol* and *salmeterol*. They are sometimes termed sympathomimetics in that they mimic the action of the sympathetic nervous system. These drugs are indicated for asthma and chronic obstructive airway disease. There are a few other drugs that are less selective but their use is cautioned in the BNF, so they have not been included here.

The autonomic nervous system controls the muscle tone in the bronchioles, allowing them to constrict and dilate. Parasympathetic nerves innervate the bronchial smooth muscle which causes bronchoconstriction. Sympathetic nerves are few in the lungs but activation of the sympathetic system causes the adrenals to release the circulatory hormone adrenaline. This binds to β_2 adrenergic (adrenaline) receptors on the smooth muscle cells of the bronchiole walls, causing the muscle

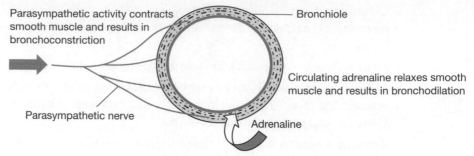

Parasympathetic activity contracts smooth muscle and results in bronchoconstriction

Bronchiole

Circulating adrenaline relaxes smooth muscle and results in bronchodilation

Parasympathetic nerve

Adrenaline

Figure 9.7 The action of parasympathetic nerves and adrenaline on the bronchioles.

cells to relax and the bronchioles to dilate (Figure 9.7). This is part of the suite of responses initiated by sympathetic activity and allows more air (and oxygen) to be drawn into the lungs during 'fight or flight' situations.

Selective beta$_2$ agonists such as **salbutamol** and **terbutaline** mimic the action of adrenaline but are selective for the beta$_2$ adrenaline receptors that occur mainly on the smooth muscle of the bronchioles. The effect of adrenaline or an agonist of adrenaline binding to these receptors causes the smooth muscle to relax and the bronchioles to dilate. Air can more easily move in and out of the lungs and so the feeling of breathlessness is relieved (Figure 9.8).

Most of the selective beta$_2$ agonists can be delivered by a self-administered, **metered dose inhaler** that delivers a predetermined quantity of the drug directly into the lungs. These drugs can also be delivered by a **nebuliser**, a face-mask adapted for drug delivery that converts a solution of the drug into an aerosol mist. **Salbutamol** and **terbutaline** are recommended for patients with an acute exacerbation of asthma and nebulisers can deliver higher doses of these drugs than can inhalers. In specific cases selective beta$_2$ agonists can be administered by tablet, syrup or injection.

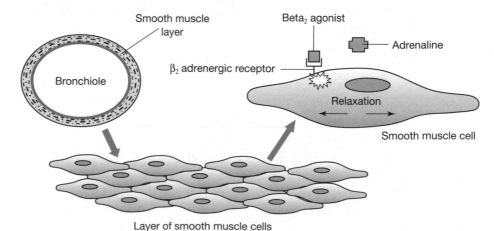

Smooth muscle layer

Beta$_2$ agonist

Adrenaline

β_2 adrenergic receptor

Bronchiole

Relaxation

Smooth muscle cell

Layer of smooth muscle cells

Figure 9.8 Beta$_2$ agonists such as **salbutamol**, mimic adrenaline and cause relaxation of bronchiolar smooth muscle, resulting in bronchodilation.

Side-effects The side-effects of selective beta$_2$ agonists are mainly due to them interacting with other adrenergic receptors. Beta$_1$ receptors on the heart can be inadvertently targeted and result in tachycardia or palpitations. Binding to beta$_2$ receptors on the skeletal muscle cells can result in fine tremor.

IN PRACTICE

Inhaled bronchodilators are generally less likely to cause side-effects than will oral or parenteral delivery. Smaller doses can be administered because the drugs are delivered directly to their target in the lungs.

Bronchodilators 2: antimuscarinic bronchodilators

There are two drugs in this group - *ipratropium bromide* and *tiotropium*. These drugs are antagonists that block muscarinic acetylcholine receptors on the smooth muscle cells of the bronchioles. Parasympathetic activity increases muscle tone in the bronchioles and so effectively acts as a bronchoconstrictor. Using an antagonist drug to block the muscarinic receptors from the effects of acetylcholine, results in bronchodilation (Figure 9.9).

One of the most common side-effects of the antimuscarinic bronchodilators is dry mouth. Parasympathetic activity stimulates digestive processes including salivation, so one effect of inhibiting the parasympathetic system is to reduce the production of saliva.

CASE STUDY

Heidi, an asthmatic 5 year old, is brought to A&E in obvious respiratory distress. She is having difficulty breathing and her mother says that she has never had such a severe asthma attack. What should be done?

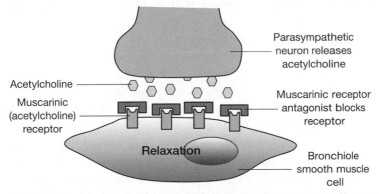

Figure 9.9 The action of a muscarinic antagonist on the smooth muscle cells of the bronchioles.

Comment on case study This is an emergency and needs immediate attention. There is no point trying to assess Heidi's lung function with a peak flow meter because, if she is unable to breathe properly, she will not be able to blow into the device. Heidi should be given supplementary oxygen and *salbutamol* or *terbutaline*, possibly delivered by a **nebuliser** until she stabilises and is able to breathe by herself.

Bronchodilators 3: *Theophylline* and *aminophylline*

Theophylline is related to caffeine and acts as a bronchodilator but its mechanism of action is not fully understood although it probably involves the relaxation of smooth muscle in the bronchioles. It can inhibit both early and late phase response and can also be used as an adjunct to β_2 agonists. *Aminophylline* is a combination of **theophylline** and **ethylenediamine**.

Theophylline has a very small window between the therapeutic dose and toxicity and both hepatic impairment and smoking can affect plasma concentration markedly. *Theophylline* interacts with drugs such as antibacterials, calcium channel blockers, diuretics and many others – see the BNF (Appendix 1).

Drug group 2: corticosteroids

Inhaled anti-inflammatory corticosteroids include **beclometasone**, **budesonide**, **ciclesonide**, **fluticasone** and **mometasone**. **Prednisolone** may be given orally in certain cases.

Anti-inflammatory corticosteroids are related to natural **glucocorticoids** which are stress hormones secreted by the adrenal gland and include **hydrocortisone** and **corticosterone**. When released during stress they increase the levels of glucose and lipids in the blood, as well as promoting the breakdown of protein. They also reduce inflammation and act as immunosuppressants, and it is these characteristics that make them desirable for therapeutic purposes. Glucocorticoids are steroids, derivatives of cholesterol and therefore lipid in nature. As such, they are able to traverse the cell membrane and exert their effect by binding to intracellular receptors, deep within the cell itself. Not all of their actions are fully understood but it is believed that their anti-inflammatory and immuno-suppressive action is due mainly to the inhibition of the release of **cytokines** (cell-signalling molecules) such as **interleukins** and **tumour necrosis factor alpha** (TNF-α). We know that mast cells and eosinophils play a part in the inflammation and sensitisation of asthmatic airways and it is believed that corticosteroids inhibit the activity of these cells. This reduces inflammation and also represses eosinophil activity, giving the body's repair mechanisms the opportunity to restore the integrity of the endothelial lining of the airways.

Anti-inflammatory corticosteroids usually include the other actions of glucocorticoids as side-effects such as an increase in blood glucose, a decrease in protein metabolism and immunosuppression. The prolonged use of orally administered corticosteroids is associated with problems such as osteoporosis, an increased risk of diabetes and the suppression of growth – which could be a real problem for children with chronic inflammatory diseases. Fortunately, inhaled corticosteroids produce far fewer side-effects than with oral administration, especially if the asthma can be controlled with only moderate dosages. Oral candidiasis can be a problem with inhaled glucocorticoids because they produce localised immuno-suppression, promoting infection from opportunistic pathogens such as the yeast, *Candida albicans*.

Asthma preventers: miscellaneous

Sodium cromoglycate and *nedocromil sodium* are useful prophylactics against exercise-induced asthma. Their mechanism of action is uncertain.

Leukotriene receptor antagonists such as *zafirlukast* and *montelukast* block leukotriene receptors in the bronchioles. Leukotrienes are produced in inflammation and blocking their receptors has been shown to induce bronchodilation. They are not used as short-term bronchodilators and are somewhat less effective than other drugs such as *salbutamol* and the corticosteroids. However, as they have an additive effect they can be useful when used in combination with other drugs.

Cough

Coughs may result from temporary upper respiratory infections or they may be a symptom of a more serious underlying disorder. In the latter case it is recommended that the main pathology is addressed before suppressing the cough. In COPD such as chronic bronchitis, cough suppressants may provide relief from cough but **sputum** retention can be a problem and increase the risk of infection. Smoker's cough is best treated by giving up smoking.

Two drugs are recommended for a dry or painful cough - *codeine phosphate* and *pholcodine*. Both are opiates and work by a poorly defined suppressive action on the 'cough centre' in the brainstem. When taken in larger doses, side-effects include constipation and respiratory depression.

Expectorants are medicines that promote the expulsion of bronchial secretions. There are many proprietary expectorant preparations and cough remedies available OTC, containing a range of drugs in various combinations but evidence for their efficacy is poor.

A QUICK RECAP on drugs used in the treatment of respiratory disorders

- There are two principal approaches to treating asthma and COPD. Bronchodilators open the airways, making breathing easier. Asthma-preventing drugs such as corticosteroids reduce inflammation, mucus production and oedema.

- Selective beta$_2$ agonists such as *salbutamol* and *terbutaline* mimic adrenaline and cause smooth muscle in the bronchioles to relax - and the bronchioles to dilate.

- Antimuscarinic bronchodilators such as *ipratropium bromide* block acetylcholine receptors and cause smooth muscle in the bronchioles to relax - and the bronchioles to dilate.

- Corticosteroids such as **beclometasone** act as immunosuppressants and reduce activity of mast cells and eosinophils that cause inflammation and long-term damage to the lining of the airways.

- Severe dry cough can be treated using **codeine**-based drugs, but suppressing a cough is not always desirable in COPD due to sputum retention.

RUNNING WORDS

Here are some of the technical terms that were included in this chapter. Read through them one by one and tick them off when you are sure that you understand them.

Allergens p. 215
Alveolar macrophages p. 213
Alveoli p. 210
Asthma p. 208
Asthma attack p. 215
Bronchi p. 211
Bronchioles p. 211
Bronchitis p. 208
Bronchospasm p. 215
Bronchus p. 211
Chemoreceptors p. 214
Chronic obstructive pulmonary disease (COPD) p. 208
Cilia p. 213
Compliance p. 212
Corticosterone p. 222
Cystic fibrosis p. 208
Cytokines p. 222
Diaphragm p. 212

Diffusion gradient p. 211
Diphtheria p. 215
Dry cough p. 218
Dyspnoea p. 216
Emphysema p. 208
Eosinophils p. 216
Epithelial cells p. 213
Expectorants p. 223
Expectoration p. 217
Expiration p. 212
External intercostals p. 212
Gas exchange p. 210
Glucocorticoids p. 222
Goblet cells p. 213
Hydrocortisone p. 222
Hypertrophy p. 217
Hypoxic drive p. 214
Inspiration p. 212
Interleukins p. 222

Internal intercostals p. 212
Late phase response p. 216
Leukotriene receptor antagonists p. 223
Lumen p. 217
Measles p. 215
Metered dose inhaler p. 220
Mucus p. 212
Nebuliser p. 220
Peak flow meter p. 217
Pneumonia p. 208
Polio p. 215
Respiratory membrane p. 211
Sputum p. 223
Tumour necrosis factor alpha (TNF-α) p. 222

REFERENCES AND FURTHER RECOMMENDED READING

All recommended websites are open access (but free registration is sometimes required).

British Lung Foundation – http://www.lunguk.org/

NICE Guidelines on COPD – http://www.nice.org.uk/guidance/CG12

NHS Website (asthma) – http://www.nhs.uk/conditions/asthma/

Your turn to try

Now you have finished reading through this chapter try answering these questions to see how much you have learned.

The answers to these questions are at the end of the book on page 286.

1 List the airways through which air flows from the mouth to the alveoli.

2 What is the average area of the alveoli? (Square metres or tennis courts will do.)

3 What happens to the rate and depth of breathing as carbon dioxide levels rise?

4 Where are the central chemoreceptors located?

5 Explain the term *hypoxic drive*.

6 What is the normal function of mucus in the airways?

7 Name five possible triggers of an asthma attack.

8 What is dyspnoea?

9 Explain the key difference between emphysema and bronchitis.

10 What is the main causative agent of emphysema and bronchitis?

11 Which cells are targeted by both **salbutamol** and **ipratropium bromide**?

12 What receptor is the main target for **ipratropium bromide**?

13 How are corticosteroids useful in asthma?

14 Why would long-term systemic use of corticosteroids be problematical in children?

15 What common side-effect might be caused by a cough reliever such as **codeine**?

Answers to questions on page 209

1 The trachea.
2 Oxygen.
3 Air enters the lungs.
4 The alveoli.
5 The pleural membranes.

Chapter 10

Disorders and drugs of the endocrine system

AIMS

By the time you have finished the chapter you should be able to understand . . .

1 The **physiology** – the structure and function of the endocrine system, especially the regulation of blood glucose, the function of the thyroid gland and the hormonal regulation of the female reproductive cycle
2 The **pathology** – disorders and pathologies associated with the endocrine system including diabetes, osteoporosis, post-menopausal symptoms and thyroid disorders
3 The **pharmacology** – the action of the major drug groups used in the treatment of key endocrine disorders and also for contraceptive purposes

CONTENTS

This chapter is organised slightly differently from previous chapters. Normally we would discuss the physiology of a system, followed by its disorders and finally the drugs used to treat those disorders. The endocrine system, however, is not a tightly integrated system like the nervous system. The various hormones discussed in this chapter, although contributing to general homeostasis, are not closely related and control different physiological processes. As a consequence, their associated pathologies affecting blood glucose, bone, reproduction and thyroid function also have very little in common (other than being associated with the endocrine system). Therefore, to make this chapter more coherent, we will group the pathologies and drugs into separate, discrete topics.

As usual, the chapter contains some brief case studies and finishes off with self-test questions to enable you to ensure that you have understood the physiology of the endocrine system, associated disorders and the pharmacology of drugs used to treat those disorders. The chapter also discusses one of the most commonly prescribed groups of drugs in the UK – hormonal contraceptives.

IN PRACTICE

Whatever your branch of clinical practice, you will undoubtedly encounter patients who have been prescribed drugs that act on the endocrine system. Some of these patients will suffer from diabetes, a disease that affects at least 2.5 million people in the UK. You may come into contact with these patients for reasons other than their diabetes, but it is still important to understand both the disease and the associated drugs to avoid potential problems such as drug interactions. Hormonal contraceptives are another common group of drugs that could be prescribed to any woman of child-bearing age. Closely related are drugs used as **hormone replacement therapy** (HRT) for older women for the treatment of post-menopausal symptoms. Again it is important to understand their action as there is the possibility that their effectiveness may be compromised by other drugs – with obvious and unfortunate consequences where they are prescribed for contraceptive purposes! As hormonal contraceptives can also have an effect on blood clotting, you need to appreciate that certain surgical procedures require them to be discontinued before the procedure can go ahead.

Introduction

The endocrine system and the nervous system together coordinate and control most physiological processes in the body. In Chapter 11 we will examine drugs prescribed for disorders of the nervous system, specifically for patients with mental health problems. In this chapter we will discuss drugs that help patients with endocrine disorders.

There are a variety of problems that can affect the glands of the endocrine system and most of these disorders result in either the over-production or under-production of the hormone normally secreted by that gland, and this can have serious consequences for homeostasis. For example, diseases of the **thyroid gland** can result in **hyperthyroidism**, where circulating levels of thyroid hormone are abnormally high or **hypothyroidism**, where circulating levels of thyroid hormone are abnormally low. The **pancreas** is another gland that can be affected by diseases that reduce the release of **insulin** – a causative factor in **diabetes**. The ovaries secrete the steroid hormones **oestrogen** and **progesterone** that fluctuate in a monthly cycle until **menopause** around the age of 45, when levels start to decline. This can result in unpleasant symptoms such as hot flushes – unpredictable episodes of sweating, accompanied by a feeling of intense warmth.

Hormonal contraceptives are widely used by women as a safe and effective method of controlling their fertility and preventing pregnancy.

WHERE ARE WE STARTING FROM?

In this chapter we will examine the endocrine system in relation to some common diseases such as diabetes and osteoporosis as well as post-menopausal problems and thyroid disorders. We will also be examining the hormonal regulation of the female reproductive cycle to explain the action of oral contraceptives. Most people are aware that we have hormones, but what they do may be more of a mystery. Anyway, let's start off with the usual short quiz to find out how much you know before we begin:

1 What is the name of the gland that releases insulin?

_____

2 What is the function of insulin?

_____

3 Name two hormones produced by the ovaries.

_____

4 Does thyroid hormone increase or decrease metabolism?

_____

5 Which pituitary hormone stimulates the development of ovarian follicles?

_____

Answers are at the end of the chapter on page 254.

How did you do? Unless you have studied human biology recently you may have struggled with some of these questions. Hormones are rather like vitamins – most people can name them but few could accurately explain their action. If you got them all correct then well done, but don't worry if you struggled as we will deal with the physiological action of all of the hormones mentioned in the quiz later in this chapter.

10.1 Principles of endocrine control

The endocrine system complements the nervous system in controlling the body. Both systems can have a major influence on the behaviour of organs and tissues, but generally the nervous system is best suited to spontaneous actions whereas the endocrine system is most effective in the long-term control of processes. Functions where speed is essential such as sight, speech and movement are best coordinated by the nervous system while processes such as growth, reproduction and the regulation of blood glucose lend themselves to hormonal control. There is, however, close cooperation between the endocrine system and the nervous system and many tissues such as the heart and blood vessels respond to both hormonal and nervous stimulation. An example of both systems working together is the so-called 'fight or flight' response to dangerous situations, where the sympathetic nervous system is reinforced by circulating adrenaline. Some **endocrine glands,** such as the pituitary, are under the direct control of the nervous system.

The endocrine system is a collection of glands and tissues that secrete hormones into the bloodstream. These hormones circulate around the body until they come into contact with receptor proteins that are found on the cell surface and also inside cells. Many of these hormonal receptors are targets for the drugs discussed in previous chapters. When a hormone binds to its receptor it produces an effect on that cell and that effect will depend on the type of hormone, the class of receptor and the location of the cell. We examined receptors in some detail in Chapter 2 and saw that each tissue expresses its own collection of receptors and, consequently, will only respond to hormones specific to those receptors.

Table 10.1 lists some of the key hormones, especially those that have a pharmacological relevance, either because their receptors form the targets for drugs or drugs interfere with their production.

Hormones can be divided into three classes . . .

- Peptide (protein) hormones, e.g. insulin
- Steroid hormones, e.g. oestrogen and progesterone
- Amine hormones, e.g. adrenaline and thyroid hormone (thyroxine).

The mechanism of action of these different classes of hormone varies according to the hormone type.

Peptide hormones These are hydrophilic (attracted by water) and dissolve in water. From this it follows that they are lipophobic (repelled by lipids) and

Table 10.1 Selected hormones released by endocrine glands and their actions

Gland or tissue	Hormone*	Targets	Effects
Posterior pituitary	Antidiuretic hormone (ADH) – vasopressin	Kidneys and arterioles	Inhibits urine production and so conserves water. Vasoconstriction maintains blood pressure
Anterior pituitary	Follicle-stimulating hormone (FSH)	Ovaries (females) Testes (males)	Stimulates ovarian follicles in females and sperm production in males
Anterior pituitary	Luteinising hormone (LH)	Ovaries (females) Testes (males)	Causes ovulation in females and testosterone secretion in males
Ovaries	Oestrogens	Anterior pituitary Breasts Uterus	Regulates reproductive cycle. Maintains secondary sexual characteristics, etc.
Ovaries	Progesterone	Anterior pituitary Uterus	Regulates reproductive cycle. Maintains pregnancy
Thyroid	Thyroid hormone	Various tissues	Regulation of metabolic rate and promotion of body growth
Adrenal cortex	Aldosterone	Kidneys	Regulates the body's sodium balance (and therefore blood pressure)
Adrenal cortex	Cortisol	Various tissues including the liver	Release of glucose, amino acids and fatty acids into the blood
Adrenal medulla	Adrenaline (epinephrine)	Various tissues – heart, blood vessels and bronchioles	Increase in blood pressure and blood glucose, bronchodilation etc.
Pancreas	Insulin and glucagon	Various tissues – liver and fat cells	Regulation of blood glucose

* Note that this is an abbreviated list of hormones, selected because of their pharmacological relevance or because they are key to physiological systems mentioned in other chapters.

insoluble in lipids. As cell membranes are essentially lipid in nature, peptide hormones are unable to pass through the cell membrane and exert their influence on the cell by binding to receptors on the cell surface (Figure 10.1).

Steroid hormones These are all derived from cholesterol and, being lipid in nature, they are lipophilic (attracted to lipids) and pass through the cell membrane. Inside the cell steroid hormones bind to their receptors and produce an effect within the cell, often the initiation of protein synthesis (Figure 10.2). For example, testosterone stimulates the production of muscle protein (which is why synthetic steroids are sometimes used illegally by some athletes to increase their muscle bulk).

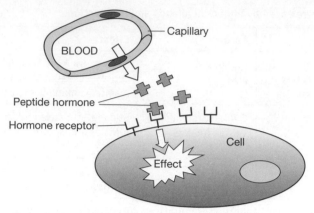

Figure 10.1 Peptide hormones bind to receptors on the surface of cells.

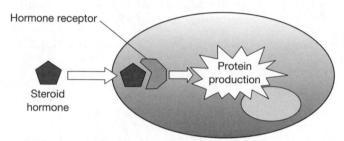

Figure 10.2 Steroid hormones bind to receptors within cells and generally initiate protein production.

Amine hormones These vary in their action. For example, adrenaline behaves as a peptide whereas thyroid hormone behaves as a steroid.

 Yes, the action of amine hormones appears contradictory but it is beyond the scope of an introductory book to explain the biochemical reason why some amines behave as peptides and others as lipids. There are plenty of more advanced books on the library shelves if you want an in-depth explanation.

 A QUICK RECAP on principles of endocrine control

- The endocrine system comprises various glands and tissues that secrete hormones into the bloodstream.

- Hormones travel in the blood and diffuse into the tissues where they bind to receptors in and on cells.

- The effect of a hormone binding to a tissue depends on the type of hormone, the class of receptor and the location of the cell.

- Hormones can be divided into three types – peptides, steroids and amines.

10.2 Disorders and drugs of the endocrine system

Diabetes

The regulation of blood glucose

Glucose, a **monosaccharide** sugar, is one of the principal fuels used by our body to make energy. In our cells, glucose is broken down to produce adenosine triphosphate (ATP), the energy-providing molecule that powers the millions of biochemical reactions that take place in our body every second.

We obtain glucose from the food we eat, predominantly starch-rich foods such as potatoes, rice, bread and pasta. In the small intestine, glucose is absorbed into the blood and routed to the liver via the hepatic portal vein. The **hepatocytes** (liver cells) absorb much of the recently acquired glucose and convert it into **glycogen**, an insoluble polymer of glucose. This is stored in the hepatocytes and can be reconverted to glucose when blood glucose levels fall.

> **Monosaccharide** literally means single sugar. Glucose is a single sugar molecule that can also exist as a disaccharide when two glucoses join to form **maltose**. Glucose molecules can also join together in long chains called polymers to form glycogen.

All cells need to make energy and most can use lipids as fuel as well as sugars. Neurons, however, rely almost exclusively on glucose for their energy, which is why the maintenance of appropriate blood glucose levels is essential for the proper functioning of the nervous system. In **hypoglycaemia** (low blood glucose levels) neurological processes in the brain can be compromised. At some time, most of us will have missed a meal and experienced the effects of low blood glucose, a feeling of being light headed along with an inability to concentrate normally. **Hyperglycaemia** (high blood glucose levels) can also cause neurological disturbance such as blurred vision and headache. Chronic hyperglycaemia, a common feature of **diabetes mellitus**, can be a contributory factor to atherosclerosis, eye problems and renal failure.

Our blood glucose levels are liable to fluctuation because our food intake can vary greatly over a 24-hour period. After meals, the body absorbs nutrients from the digestive system and, though buffered somewhat by glucose storage in the liver, blood glucose levels rise. When digestion is complete and nutrient absorption tails off, blood glucose levels fall. Despite these fluctuations, the body needs to maintain blood glucose levels within certain limits. The brain is especially sensitive to falls in blood glucose as it relies solely on glucose for its energy and has very little glucose storage capacity of its own. Typical fasting levels of blood glucose lie between 3.3 and 6.1 mmol/l and results outside this range could indicate a dysfunction in glucose regulation such as occurs in diabetes mellitus.

IN PRACTICE

Fasting blood glucose levels are used to determine whether a person may have diabetes as they are more reliable than random blood tests which may be more of an indication of recent eating patterns. Generally a fasting glucose level in excess of 7.0 mmol/l indicates a strong possibility that the individual is diabetic.

The pancreas

The pancreas is a large gland that nestles under the stomach and plays an important part in glucose regulation. The position of the pancreas relative to adjacent organs is shown in Figure 10.3. The pancreas has a dual role, secreting both digestive enzymes into the duodenum via the pancreatic duct and also releasing insulin and **glucagon**, the two key hormones in glucose regulation, into the blood. These two hormones are released from small clusters of glandular cells called the **Islets of Langerhans**.

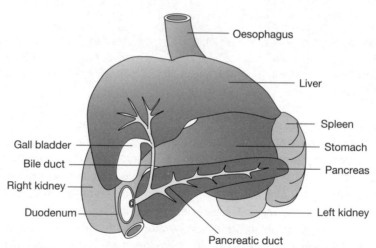

Figure 10.3 The position of the pancreas relative to adjacent organs. (Note that the pancreas is shown in front of the stomach here for illustrative purposes.)

How the body responds to an increase in blood glucose

After a meal the resulting increase in blood glucose is detected by the β (beta) cells of the pancreatic islets causing them to release more insulin into the blood. Insulin stimulates cells, especially **adipose** (fat cells) and muscle cells, to take up glucose from the blood. Glucose is a relatively large molecule and to enter cells it requires transmembrane **glucose transporters**. When insulin binds to insulin receptors, cells are stimulated to increase the numbers of glucose transporters in the cell membrane, a process called **translocation** (Figure 10.4). The more transporters that are recruited, the more glucose is transported into cells – with a corresponding drop in blood glucose.

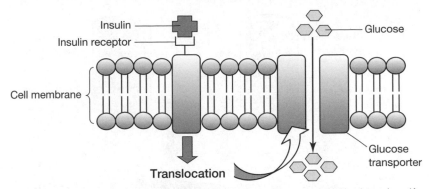

Figure 10.4 The binding of insulin to insulin receptors causes the translocation of glucose transporters to the cell membrane and this promotes the uptake of glucose from the blood.

> **Translocation** - glucose transporters in the cytoplasm of the cell are moved and inserted into the cell membrane so that glucose can enter through them into the cell.

Insulin also has other effects on the body's cells, all of which contribute to an increase in glucose usage and storage - and therefore a reduction in blood glucose.

> **KEY FACT**
> When blood glucose levels rise, the body releases more insulin that allows cells to take up more glucose from the blood.

How the body responds to a decrease in blood glucose

In the hours after a meal, when digestion is complete and blood glucose and insulin levels fall, this causes the α (alpha) cells of the pancreas to release the hormone glucagon. Glucagon has the opposite effect to insulin in that it increases blood glucose levels and promotes processes that spare glucose usage. Glucagon works primarily on hepatocytes to convert stored glycogen into glucose and release it into the blood. A summary of the contrasting actions of glucagon and insulin is shown in Figure 10.5.

REALITY CHECK

Can you explain the difference between glucose, glycogen and glucagon?

Disorders of blood glucose regulation: diabetes mellitus

This very common disease is found in two main forms - Type 1 and Type 2 diabetes, both of which are increasing annually in the UK. Type 2 diabetes is the most common form, accounting for around 90 per cent of diabetes. It is primarily a disease of affluent societies although ironically it is more common among people of lower

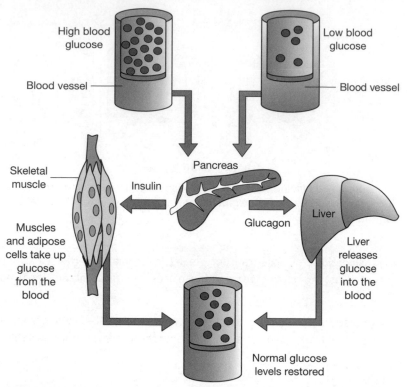

Figure 10.5 Summary of the actions of insulin and glucagon in the regulation of blood glucose.

economic status where obesity, one of the key risk factors for diabetes, is most widespread. A family history of diabetes can also be a predisposing factor for diabetes and people of Asian and Afro-Caribbean origin are also at greater risk. Diabetes is fundamentally a disease involving dysfunctions in glucose regulation, but despite it being such a common disease and much research having been undertaken, the mechanisms underlying the problem are by no means fully understood. However, as our knowledge of these diseases improves, so does the possibility for advances in treatment or even a cure.

Type 1 diabetes is primarily a disease of the young and is the result of an auto-immune destruction of the insulin-producing β cells of the pancreas. Insulin production is severely compromised and regular insulin injections are necessary to regulate blood glucose.

Type 2 diabetes was once a disease of middle age but with an increase in childhood obesity, many younger people are now developing the disease. It is thought that an increase in the consumption of sugar-rich foods is primarily responsible. This causes a long-term elevation of insulin levels and as a consequence, tissues become resistant to the action of insulin and eventually insulin production itself declines. These two factors result in hyperglycaemia because the mechanism that allows glucose to enter cells has become compromised. Dietary modification may be sufficient to control Type 2 diabetes initially but many sufferers progress to require antidiabetic drugs and insulin injections.

In both forms of diabetes mellitus, abnormally high levels of blood glucose are encountered, typically over 11 mmol/l. This can overwhelm glucose reabsorption in the kidneys, causing it to appear in the urine, a condition called **glycosuria**. Other symptoms of diabetes include an increase in thirst, an increase in urine production and lethargy.

> **DID YOU KNOW . . .** that the word mellitus has its origin in the Latin word *mel*, meaning honey? Diabetes can result in glucose appearing in the urine, making it sweet, and in days gone by physicians tested for diabetes by tasting their patient's urine. Be thankful for modern testing methods!

In Type 1 diabetes, **ketosis** may also be encountered. Ironically, this is caused by cells being starved of glucose. Remember that cells need insulin in order to obtain glucose from the blood so, in the absence of insulin, there is an abundance of glucose in the blood while the cells themselves are starved of this essential energy molecule. In an effort to maintain energy production, cells switch to lipids as their main source of fuel, resulting in the production of **ketones** as a by-product which, being acidic, can cause **ketoacidosis**. Diabetes can be the cause or contributory factor of many other chronic pathologies including **nephropathy** (disease of the kidneys), **retinopathy** (disease of the retina) and cardiovascular disease.

> **CASE STUDY**
>
> Kulvinder is a bright 9-year-old girl who developed Type 1 diabetes when she was 8. Her mother had noticed that Kulvinder seemed tired and listless and was drinking more fluids than usual. Her auntie had developed Type 2 diabetes when she was 45 and Kulvinder's mother was worried that diabetes might be a problem for the family. Is it likely that there was a genetic link between her auntie's Type 2 diabetes and Kulvinder's Type 1 diabetes?

Comment of case study It is unlikely that there is any genetic link between Kulvinder's Type I diabetes and her auntie's Type 2 diabetes because they are two distinct diseases with different causes. However, there could be a genetic predisposition for both diseases in the family, meaning that there is a greater risk for family members. There is little that can be done to predict or prevent Type 1 diabetes because it is an autoimmune disease. However, lifestyle can have an influence on the development of Type 2 diabetes, so family members would do well to ensure that they have a healthy diet, take plenty of exercise and keep their weight within recommended limits.

Drugs used in the treatment of diabetes mellitus

There are two approaches to the treatment of diabetes. The normal treatment for Type 1 diabetes is insulin given by subcutaneous injection. This is to replace the body's own insulin deficiency where endogenous insulin production is minimal or non-existent. Treatment for Type 2 diabetes is more complex because this form of the disease can vary in its intensity and nature. Oral antidiabetic drugs work by a variety of means, generally either stimulating residual insulin secretion by the β cells of the pancreas, or encouraging muscle and adipose cells to take up glucose from the blood. Supplementary insulin may also be required by some Type 2 diabetics.

IN PRACTICE

Before Type 2 diabetics are prescribed oral antidiabetic drugs, control of the disease is usually attempted by at least three months of dietary modification and an increase in exercise. Eating complex carbohydrates that release their sugars slowly can help to maintain stable blood glucose levels. Exercise increases the cellular uptake of glucose.

There are various types of insulin available for injection. All of these are the result of many years of research and development, stretching back to the 1920s when insulin, extracted from the pancreases of cattle, was first used to treat diabetic patients. Modern insulins are from three sources – modified **porcine** (pig), **bovine** (cattle) or **genetically engineered** human insulin. The latter form of human insulin is not extracted from humans but is produced in bacteria and yeast using genetic engineering. The gene that codes for human insulin is inserted into bacteria and yeast, which produce the insulin protein in large quantities. The protein produced in this way requires further purification and modification before it can be used as a medicine. The advantage of human insulin is that it is self-evidently more similar in structure to the patient's own insulin so there is less chance of it causing an adverse reaction.

Insulin can be further modified to affect the rate at which it is absorbed, thus delaying the time of onset and prolonging the duration of its effect. This modification is effected by attaching zinc or other residues to the insulin molecule or by genetically engineering insulins with a slightly different amino acid sequence. The various insulins currently available are categorised by the rate at which they begin to act and the duration of their action.

● **Short-acting insulins** have a rapid onset (30 to 60 minutes), a peak action of between 2 to 4 hours with duration up to 8 hours. These insulins include *insulin aspart*, *insulin glulisine* and *insulin lispro*.

● **Intermediate and long-lasting insulins** have an onset of between 1 to 2 hours, a peak action of between 4 to 12 hours and duration of 16 to 35 hours. These insulins include *insulin detemir, insulin glargine, insulin zinc suspension, isophane insulin* and *protamine zinc insulin.*

● **Biphasic insulins** are a mixture of intermediate and fast-acting insulins that produce rapid onset but long-lasting effects. These insulins include *biphasic insulin aspart, biphasic insulin lispro* and *biphasic isophane insulin.*

DID YOU KNOW... that insulin has to be injected because it is a protein and proteins will not survive digestive enzymes in the gut? Inhaled insulins were introduced but subsequently withdrawn following concerns over safety. Needless to say that the inhaled insulins were popular with patients because they were needle-less!

Antidiabetic drugs

These drugs are used to treat Type 2 diabetes when dietary and exercise changes have failed to control the condition.

1 **Sulphonylureas** – Short-acting sulphonylureas include *gliclazide* and *tolbutamide*. *Chlorpropamide, glibenclamide* and *glipizide* are longer acting and may thus have more side-effects such as hypoglycaemia. *Chlorpropamide* is especially prone to causing side-effects and its use is no longer recommended. All of these drugs work by opening Ca^{2+} channels in the cell membrane of the β cells of the pancreas, stimulating them to release insulin. These drugs are only suitable for use in Type 2 diabetes where the β cells retain some insulin-secreting capacity.

2 **Biguanides** – *Metformin hydrochloride* is the only biguanide currently available. It works by increasing the uptake of glucose by cells but only where there is a residual production of insulin by the pancreas.

3 *Acarbose* inhibits the **α-glucosidase** enzymes in the gut that have a role in the digestion of starches. This reduces the rate at which starches are broken down and consequently the rate at which glucose is absorbed. This can reduce the risk of hyperglycaemia after a meal. Unfortunately, undigested sugars in the gut can feed gas-producing bacteria resulting in flatulence, a side-effect that (not surprisingly) puts off many patients from continuing with this drug.

4 *Exenatide* is a recently introduced drug which increases insulin secretion while reducing glucagon release by the α cells of the pancreas and slowing the rate of gastric emptying. It is a synthetic form of **exendin-4**, a hormone first isolated from the saliva of an American desert lizard. Exendin-4 mimics the action of **glucagon-like peptide-1** of the **incretin** family of peptides, released by the gastrointestinal tract immediately following a meal (Figure 10.6). As it relies on residual activity of the pancreatic β cells, it is only licensed for the treatment of Type 2 diabetes.

5 *Sitagliptin* is another recently introduced drug that works in the same pathways described above for *exenatide*. *Sitagliptin* is an inhibitor of **dipeptidylpeptidase-4**, an enzyme that breaks down the **incretins**. By blocking dipeptidylpeptidase-4, *sitagliptin* increases natural incretin levels; this increases insulin production and suppresses glucagon production. As with *exenatide*, *sitagliptin* is only licensed for the treatment of Type 2 diabetes.

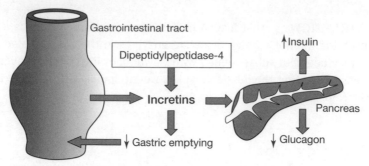

Figure 10.6 Food in the gastrointestinal tract stimulates the release of incretins that promote the secretion of insulin while inhibiting both glucagon and gastric emptying. Dipeptidylpeptidase-4 is an enzyme that breaks down incretins.

6 **Meglitinides** are currently represented by two drugs, *nateglinide* and *repaglinide*. They work by a very similar mechanism to the sulphonylureas, stimulating insulin release by pancreatic β cells in Type 2 diabetes.

7 **Thiazolidinediones** include *pioglitazone* and *rosiglitazone*. The mechanism of action of these drugs is complex and not fully understood but they appear to enhance insulin signalling in adipocytes, and thus the uptake of glucose from the blood. Concerns have been expressed recently regarding the safety of *rosiglitazone* and it is no longer recommended for patients with ischaemic heart disease or peripheral arterial disease.

Hypoglycaemia

Acute hypoglycaemia can arise from an overdose of insulin and chronic hypoglycaemia from excess endogenous insulin production. Hypoglycaemia is generally treated via the administration of glucose, but if sugar cannot be given by mouth then *glucagon* may be prescribed via injection. This stimulates the liver to convert stores of glycogen into glucose for release into the bloodstream.

A QUICK RECAP on diabetes, insulins and antidiabetic drugs

- Glucose levels in the blood need to be regulated to ensure that levels do not fall too low or rise too high.

- When glucose levels rise after a meal, the pancreas releases insulin that encourages muscle and fat cells to take up glucose from the blood.

- When glucose levels fall between meals, the pancreas releases glucagon that stimulates the liver to release glucose to increase blood sugar levels

- Type 1 diabetes is an auto-immune disease that destroys the insulin-producing cells of the pancreas. Type 1 sufferers cannot produce insulin and require insulin injections.

- Type 2 diabetes usually develops later in life and may be caused by factors such as obesity. Type 2 sufferers may be able to control their diabetes by diet and drugs but sometimes insulin injections are also necessary.

- Injectable insulins are divided into short acting, intermediate and long acting, and biphasic, and vary in their time to onset and their duration.

- Antidiabetic drugs are used only for the treatment of Type 2 diabetes.

- By different mechanisms, drugs such as *exenatide, sitagliptin*, the sulphonylureas and the meglitinides, stimulate the pancreas to release insulin (where residual capacity remains).

- *Metformin* and the thiazolidinediones increase the uptake of glucose by cells.

- *Acarbose* reduces the rate at which glucose is absorbed from the gut.

Hormonal regulation of the female reproductive cycle – and associated drugs

The introduction of female hormonal contraceptives, 'the pill' in the 1960s, revolutionised sexual habits in the UK and probably changed society forever. For the first time it allowed women to take charge of their own fertility and prevented millions of unwanted pregnancies. The contraceptive pill proved to be a safe and (if used correctly) 99 per cent effective method of contraception, and although the formulations have changed somewhat over the last 40 years, the pharmacological action of the drugs is still essentially the same. These drugs have other uses besides contraception, helping to prevent painful periods and alleviating some of the post-menopausal symptoms suffered by many older women.

The 28-day female reproductive cycle produces changes in a woman's body that prepares her for conception. Over the month, the **endometrium** (the lining of the uterus) develops into a nutrient-rich structure, ready to receive the ovum that is released by the ovaries midway through the cycle. If fertilisation occurs, the fertilised ovum implants itself in the wall of the uterus and the wonderful process of embryological development starts which, in nine months' time, will result in the birth of a new human being. If the woman does not conceive during this time, the endometrium is shed in a flow of menstrual blood - a 'period'. After the period, the process starts all over again. The cycle is controlled by an intricate interplay of two hormones released by the **anterior pituitary**:

- follicle-stimulating hormone (FSH)
- luteinising hormone (LH)

and two hormones released by the ovaries:

- oestrogen
- progesterone.

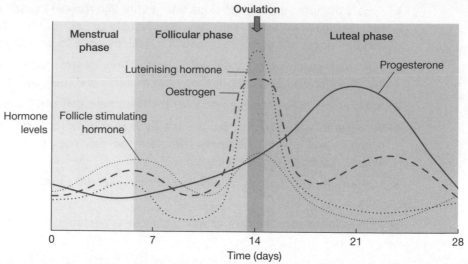

Figure 10.7 Simplified graph showing changing levels of hormones during the 28-day reproductive cycle (hormone levels are in arbitrary units).

> **Oestrogen** and **progesterone** are the common names for the two types of hormones secreted by the ovaries. There are in fact several oestrogens including oestradiol, oestriol and oestrone. Progesterone is the main circulating form of the **progestogen** group.

The cycle can be divided into three phases, as shown in Figure 10.7:

1 **The menstrual phase** – This starts on the first day of menstruation and lasts 4 to 6 days. During this phase the lining of the uterus is shed in a flow of blood.

2 **The follicular phase** – During the next 8 to 10 days, FSH promotes the development of a follicle in one of the ovaries containing the maturing ovum. As the follicle develops it starts to produce oestrogen and the amount of oestrogen steadily increases as the follicle itself enlarges. The increase in oestrogen towards the end of the follicular phase stimulates a surge in luteinising hormone (LH) that causes the follicle to release its ovum in the process, known as **ovulation**. The ovum travels from the ovary to the uterus, down the oviduct where it has the potential to be fertilised by incoming sperm.

3 **The luteal phase** – This final phase can vary considerably depending on whether the ovum is fertilised or not. If fertilisation occurs, the embryo that is implanted in the endometrium sends a hormonal signal to the ovaries. This maintains the high levels of progesterone that occur immediately after ovulation. Progesterone maintains the structural integrity of the endometrium and prevents further menstruation. If fertilisation does not occur, the progesterone levels tail off, removing support from the endometrium which is shed in the menstrual flow.

Control of the reproductive cycle involves a complex interplay between the pituitary and the ovarian hormones. As hormone levels change, this signals the pituitary and ovaries to modify the release of their hormones which brings about further changes and responses in the intricate hormone balance. Artificially changing hormone levels with synthetic oestrogens and progestogens interferes with the cycle and, as we will see later in this chapter, prevents ovulation and conception.

Postmenopausal problems and hormone replacement therapy

Around the age of 45 years, most women start to go through a phase of changes called the menopause that marks the end of their reproductive life. For a woman who has kept herself fit and healthy this may seem particularly unfair because while her partner may still be able to father children, she will be unable to conceive them. This seemingly iniquitous situation is generally thought to be an evolutionary adaptation that dates back tens of thousands of years to an era when times were tough and the average human life span was less than 40 years. Evolution is ruthless in its economy and will eliminate unnecessary expenditure, so it may well be that there was no selective advantage in the female body storing more ova than necessary for an average lifespan that was less than 40 years. Few women over that age were likely to bring a baby to term or live to look after that baby, so genes for reproductive capacity in what was then 'old age' would not be selected. On the other hand, sperm are relatively cheap on resources, so there was little selective advantage for evolution to limit their production (although sperm production does decline somewhat with age).

Evolutionary history aside, in the twenty-first century many women in their mid-forties are still in excellent physical condition and are looking forward to another 40 or more years of healthy and fruitful life. It is therefore unfortunate for these women that the menopause can be quite distressing because changes in circulating hormone levels can produce some very uncomfortable symptoms.

During the period from **menarche** (the onset of menstruation) to menopause, oestrogen levels are maintained by the activity of the oestrogen-producing **ovarian follicles**. Menopause occurs because there are a finite number of follicles in the ovaries and when they have all been through the monthly cycle of maturation and ovulation, there comes a point when their supply is exhausted. Without follicles, the supply of oestrogen relies on the adrenal glands which continue to produce some oestrogen but in a form that is less potent. Before menopause, when oestrogen levels are relatively high, these high levels have a suppressive effect on FSH and LH, and when oestrogen levels fall with menopause, FSH and LH levels rise. These changes in hormone levels contribute to the symptoms associated with menopause such as hot flushes, vaginal dryness, loss of sexual drive, mood swings, an increased susceptibility to cardiovascular disease and **osteoporosis** (thinning of the bones).

> **Ovarian follicles** are small, fluid-filled sacs containing the developing ovum that develop each month in the ovaries. Their development is stimulated by the aptly named follicle-stimulating hormone (FSH) and in the middle of the cycle, luteinising hormone (LH) triggers the ovum's release during ovulation.

Hormone replacement therapy (HRT)

As post-menopausal problems are caused as a result of falling hormone levels, the pharmacological solution is to replace these hormones artificially. Restoring hormones to pre-menopausal levels brings significant relief to many women for whom problems such as hot flushes can cause considerable distress. Many proprietary HRT preparations are available, delivering a combination of oestrogens and progesterone. Low dose oestrogens in the form of **oestradiol** are usually administered continuously with a synthetic progestogen such as **norethisterone** or **levonorgestrel** added for 12–14 days in the second half of the cycle, mimicking the hormonal environment created in the natural follicular and luteal phases. Because the regime is cyclical in nature, withdrawal bleeding may occur when the progesterone part of the course is completed. Twelve months after the last menstrual period, many women switch to a regime of continuous low-dose combined oestrogen and progesterone which relieves post-menopausal symptoms without the inconvenience of monthly bleeding.

Hormone replacement therapy may be delivered orally or via a transdermal patch. As steroid hormones, oestrogens and progestogens are readily absorbed through the skin. Progesterone itself is not suitable for oral use because it is nearly completely metabolised by first-pass metabolism in the liver (as explained in Chapter 3). This is why synthetic progestogens are used in oral contraceptives.

Tibolone acts as a combined synthetic oestrogen and progesterone and is used for the short-term treatment of post-menopausal symptoms.

Hormone replacement therapy: side-effects and dangers

Apart from the usual short-term side-effects with HRT such as nausea and vomiting, come the symptoms associated with normal cyclical changes in hormonal levels, including bloating, abdominal cramps and tenderness of the breasts – and of course the return of monthly menstruation. Unpleasant though these symptoms may be, there are long-term concerns with extending a woman's exposure to oestrogens. Specifically, there is a small but significant increase in the risk of developing breast, endometrial and ovarian cancers plus an increase in the risk of stroke and venous thrombosis. The Committee on Safety of Medicines (CSM) has published a series of reports on the safety of HRT based on evidence from clinical trials. In all cases, the increased risk, in particular with combined oestrogen and progesterone HRT, is less than 1 per cent over a five-year period and the CSM is of the opinion that the small increase in risk from HRT is outweighed by its benefits in the relief of post-menopausal symptoms. *Tibolone* also increases the risk of breast cancer but not as much as for combined HRT.

A QUICK RECAP on hormonal regulation of the female reproductive cycle and hormone replacement therapy

- The 28-day female reproductive cycle is controlled by pituitary and ovarian hormones.
- The pituitary hormone, follicle-stimulating hormone (FSH), promotes the development of the ovarian follicles and luteinising hormone (LH) promotes ovulation.
- The ovarian hormone, oestrogen, plays a part in regulating the follicular phase of the cycle and progesterone prepares the uterus for pregnancy.
- At menopause, the ovarian production of oestrogen and progesterone is curtailed.
- Falling levels of these hormones produce symptoms such as hot flushes, vaginal dryness, loss of libido and mood swings.
- Hormone replacement therapy, a mixture of oestrogens and progestogens, returns the hormonal profile to its pre-menopausal state.
- There are small additional risks with HRT of developing breast, endometrial and ovarian cancers plus an increase in the risk of stroke and venous thrombosis.

Osteoporosis

Osteoporosis is primarily a disease of old age that occasionally occurs in men but is most commonly found in post-menopausal women where a reduction in oestrogen is the main cause. Bone density reaches its peak between 20 and 30 years of age, and after that there is a steady, but initially unnoticeable, decline. This is a normal physiological ageing process but when bone density is reduced to the point where the structural integrity of the bone is compromised, it has become osteoporosis. Bone density is maintained by lifestyle as well as hormonal factors. Exercise and a good diet are key factors in keeping bones healthy. Exercise, especially impact exercise such as running, tennis and gymnastics, strengthens bones – as does a diet high in fruit, vegetables and calcium (an important component of both bones and teeth). Unfortunately, many older people do not exercise, relatively few engage in sports, poor nutrition is endemic in our society and all of this adds to their risk of developing osteoporosis.

DID YOU KNOW . . . that just walking around can strengthen bones? In the 1970s when humans first started to spend long periods in space, they discovered on their return to earth that the astronauts had lost a lot of their bone density due to months spent at zero gravity. These days, astronauts exercise while in space to stress their bones and keep them healthy.

Besides the acceleration of normal loss of bone density through ageing and menopause, there are diseases such as **hyperparathyroidism** and **thyrotoxicosis** as well as self-inflicted problems such as alcohol abuse that can exacerbate the problem. The long-term use of corticosteroids for diseases such as rheumatoid arthritis can also result in osteoporosis.

> **Hyperparathyroidism** is an excess of parathyroid hormone (PTH) released by the parathyroid glands on the posterior of the thyroid. PTH plays a key role in calcium regulation, so when its levels are elevated it causes calcium to be removed from the bones, which can lead to osteoporosis.

Before we look at the available drugs and their pharmacological action, we need to understand a little more about how bone density is maintained and how this mechanism breaks down in osteoporosis.

Bones are complex living tissue, not as some may imagine, relatively inert sections of inorganic scaffolding that support the muscles. Various cells are involved in maintaining the bone matrix but of pharmacological relevance are the **osteocytes**, **osteoblasts** and **osteoclasts**. Unlike most tissues, bone is constantly being remodelled by teams of osteoclast cells that demolish small sections of bone and by teams of osteoblast cells that rebuild it. When this process is finished, osteocyte cells are left behind, contained within the bone where their metabolic activity maintains the integrity of the **bone matrix** (Figure 10.8).

ANOTHER WAY TO PICTURE THIS

Imagine the osteoclasts and osteoblasts as teams of builders whose job it is to replace all the old bricks in a building. Osteoclasts specialise in demolition while the osteoblasts are bricklayers. If they followed each other, with the osteoclasts constantly filling in the holes left by the osteoblasts, then eventually the whole building would be replaced with new brickwork.

Osteoporosis is primarily a disease of old age and is accelerated in post-menopausal women by lower levels of circulating oestrogen. At a cellular level, the changes observed in osteoporotic bone, lower density, spongy appearance, fragility, etc., are due to changes in the activity of the cells that are involved in maintaining bone density. Essentially, there is an imbalance in activity between

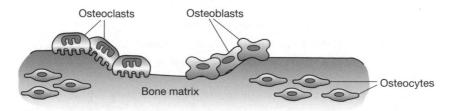

Figure 10.8 Remodelling of the bone matrix by osteoclasts and osteoblasts.

the osteoclasts and osteoblasts. Recalling our likening osteoclasts to a demolition team and osteoblasts to bricklayers, you can imagine the situation that would develop if the demolition team carried on working while the bricklayers went on strike. This is effectively what happens in osteoporosis. The post-menopausal fall in oestrogen levels only slightly affects osteoclasts, but it causes osteoblast activity to decline significantly. With the normal balance between these two groups of cells interrupted, bone building fails to keep up with bone demolition and eventually the bone matrix becomes spongy and fragile, leading to an increased risk of fractures – from even minor bumps and falls.

> **Bone matrix** is the non-cellular part of the bone that gives bone its strength and rigidity. It comprises inorganic calcium phosphate embedded in a connective tissue called collagen. The calcium phosphate gives the bone its hardness and the collagen makes it tough and resistant to breakage.

There are drugs available to help with osteoporosis but ideally it should be prevented by individuals adopting a lifestyle that keeps bones healthy. Ideally, women should try to maximise their bone density prior to menopause by regular impact exercise such as aerobics or jogging and adopting a healthy diet with foods containing plenty of calcium and vitamin D – the vitamin essential for the efficient absorption of calcium from food. Going into menopause with strong bones and maintaining a healthy lifestyle after menopause is undoubtedly the best way of delaying the onset of this disease.

Where drug treatment is deemed necessary for osteoporosis, the bisphosphonates are the drugs of choice, in particular, *alendronic acid*, *disodium etidronate* and *risedronate sodium*. *Ibandronic acid* and *strontium ranelate* are also licensed for osteoporosis but are not recommended for general use.

The bisphosphonates have an affinity for calcium and so are naturally absorbed into the bone matrix. During the remodelling process, the osteoclasts absorb the bone and so take up the bisphosphonates. This induces **apoptosis** in the osteoclasts, a form of cell suicide, and so the balance of remodelling shifts back to the bone-builders, the osteoblasts, and this helps to maintain bone density (Figure 10.9).

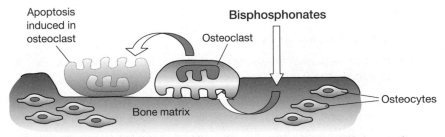

Figure 10.9 Bisphosphonates absorbed into the bone matrix are taken up by osteoclasts inducing apoptosis.

> **Apoptosis** is programmed cell death, a form of 'cell suicide'. The cell is induced to die in a controlled manner either by external or internal signals. This is very useful in multicellular organisms because cancerous or virally infected cells can be eliminated before the problem spreads.

Other drugs for osteoporosis

Although the bisphosphonates are the main drugs used for the treatment of osteoporosis, another approach is to increase circulating oestrogen levels and so slow the rate of bone loss. Hormone replacement therapy has been discussed above, and although it is effective for helping with post-menopausal symptoms, it is not generally recommended as a first-line treatment for osteoporosis.

Calcitonin and **parathyroid hormone** (PTH) are also licensed for treating osteoporosis. These are hormones involved in calcium balance released by the parathyroid glands that are found on the posterior of the thyroid gland itself. Calcitonin is responsible for conserving bone and it does this by inhibiting osteoclast activity. In drug form, the calcitonin used is synthetic or recombinant salmon calcitonin, *salcaltonin*, and it is also used in the prophylaxis of osteoporosis in patients who may suffer long periods of immobilisation. Parathyroid hormone is an unlikely candidate to be recommended as an anti-osteoporotic drug because PTH normally promotes bone reabsorption by osteoclasts. This leads to an increase in blood calcium levels at the expense of bone, and chronically high levels of PTH (as found in hyperparathyroidism) can result in osteoporosis. However, the **pulsatile** release of PTH has the opposite effects and promotes osteoblast activity, which is why daily subcutaneous injections of PTH give the fluctuations in levels that tip the balance towards bone formation and help to increase bone density. *Teriparatide* is a relatively recent recombinant form of PTH that as been licensed to treat osteoporosis.

DID YOU KNOW . . . that low body weight is also a risk factor for osteoporosis, and that being overweight can stress the bones and make them stronger? Unfortunately, obesity is also a risk factor for cardiovascular disease and diabetes, so if you want to keep your bones and your heart healthy, reach for your running shoes rather than the cream cakes!

A QUICK RECAP on osteoporosis

- Post-menopausal women are particularly susceptible to osteoporosis because of reduced levels of oestrogen, a hormone that supports bone formation.
- Bones are constantly being remodelled by the balanced activity of osteoclasts (bone breakers) and osteoblasts (bone makers).
- In osteoporosis, the balance swings towards the osteoclasts and bones become weaker.

- Bisphosphonates induce apoptosis (cell death) in osteoclasts.
- Calcitonin and parathyroid hormone are used as drugs, mimicking natural hormones to swing the balance of osteoclast and osteoblast activity towards bone formation.

Oral contraceptives

Oral contraceptives are popular methods of preventing pregnancy. They are divided into three categories, the most popular of which is the combined oral contraceptive, a mixture of oestrogens and progestogens. Progestogen-only contraceptives are generally reserved for use immediately after birth or prior to elective surgery. As oestrogen interferes with lactation, it is unsuitable if the mother is breast feeding. It is also recommended that combined hormonal contraceptives be discontinued four weeks prior to major elective surgery, surgery to the legs and surgery that involves immobilisation of the lower limbs. This is because oestrogen has a pro-thrombotic effect and could cause venous thromboembolism.

Oral contraceptives work mainly by suppressing the release of the two pituitary hormones LH and FSH. This inhibits the development of the ovarian follicle and prevents ovulation. Essentially, the body is responding to levels of oestrogens and progestogens that normally equate to pregnancy (where ovulation is suppressed), and if the ovum is not released, fertilisation and conception cannot occur.

Combined hormonal contraceptives contain an oestrogen and a progestogen. The oestrogen is commonly **ethinyloestradiol** and the progestogen may be *norethisterone*, *levonorgestrel*, *gestodene*, *norgestimate* or *desogestrel*. There is typically a 5:1 ratio progestogen to oestrogen. The course of oral contraceptives normally lasts for 21 days and after the final pill in the course, the circulating levels of oestrogen and progesterone fall and withdrawal bleeding occurs, mimicking a menstrual period.

The oestrogen in combined oral contraceptives suppresses FSH release and follicle development is inhibited. The progestogen component of the pill suppresses LH, and ovulation is inhibited. Additionally, the progestogen thickens the cervical mucus making it inhospitable to sperm, and preventing them from reaching the uterus. The development and maturation of endometrium is also inhibited by the progestogens, which discourages the implantation of any fertilised egg.

Unwanted effects of combined contraceptives include fluid retention, weight gain, nausea, vomiting, headache, breast tenderness, etc. See the BNF for a full list of potential side-effects.

The use of oral contraceptives may result in a small increase in the risk of thromboembolism, breast cancer and hypertension in certain individuals, depending on age, family history and lifestyle. There is, however, a corresponding protective effect against ovarian and endometrial cancers. Pregnancy itself is also a risk factor that must be weighed against the small risks presented by this relatively secure form of contraception.

There are interactions with other drugs that can reduce the effectiveness of the combined contraceptives. These include *rifampicin, rifabutin, carbamazepine, griseofulvin, phenytoin* and the herbal antidepressant, St John's wort (see BNF for full list). All of these, but especially *rifampicin* and *rifabutin*, induce hepatic enzyme activity that causes hormonal contraceptives to be metabolised more quickly, lowering their blood concentration levels – with obvious and possibly unfortunate consequences. Broad spectrum antibiotics, such as *ampicillin*, have a similar effect but by a different mechanism.

Progestogen-only contraceptives

Although this group has a higher failure rate than combined contraceptives, they provide an alternative form of oral contraception when oestrogen is contraindicated. For example, they are suitable for women undergoing elective surgery because they are less likely to cause clotting than would oestrogen. Those women at risk from cardiovascular disease such as heavy smokers, diabetics and sufferers from hypertension can also be prescribed progestogen-only contraceptives in preference to the oestrogen-containing combined pill. Immediately after childbirth they are useful because, unlike oestrogen, they do not interfere with lactation. Examples include preparations containing *norethisterone, levonorgestrel, desogestrel* and *etynodiol diacetate*.

The effect of progestogen-only contraceptives on ovulation is variable and their main contraceptive effect is the thickening of cervical mucus, making it inhospitable to sperm. It may also make the endometrium less susceptible to implantation by the fertilised ovum.

Emergency or post-coital contraception

This is a single high dose of *levonorgestrel* taken as soon as possible within the three days after unprotected sexual intercourse.

Its main actions are the inhibition of ovulation and possibly the prevention of implantation. Emergency contraception is distinct from chemical abortion because the *levonorgestrel* has no effect on established pregnancies.

A QUICK RECAP on oral contraceptives

- Combined hormonal contraceptives contain an oestrogen and a progestogen that raise hormone levels, similar to those in pregnancy.

- This suppresses LH and FSH release, therefore follicle development and ovulation are both inhibited. As the ovum is not released, fertilisation cannot take place.

- Many drugs such as *rifampicin* and *rifabutin* interact with combined contraceptives and reduce their effectiveness.

- Progestogen-only contraceptives are useful after childbirth and before elective surgery. Their primary action is the thickening of cervical mucus.

- Emergency contraception involves a large dose of *levonorgestrel* that inhibits ovulation.

The thyroid gland: physiology, pathology and associated drugs

The thyroid is quite a large gland situated in the neck, in front of the trachea and just below the **thyroid cartilage**, a protuber-ance in men known as the 'Adam's apple'. In shape the thyroid consists of two lobes and looks rather like a butterfly (Figure 10.10).

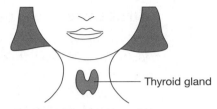

Thyroid gland

Figure 10.10 Location of the thyroid gland.

The thyroid releases various hormones, the most pharmacologically important ones being **thyroxine** (T_4) and the more active **triiodothyronine** (T_3). Thyroxine T_4 has a much longer half life than T_3 and is the main circulating thyroid hormone. However, T_4 has relatively weak activity and is effectively a **pro-hormone** because before it becomes active it has to be con-verted to T_3 inside the cells of the body. Iodine is an essential component of both of these hormones and over 99.9 per cent of the body's iodine is concentrated in the thyroid gland. The release of the thyroid hormones is controlled by **thyroid-stimulating hormone** (TSH) released by the anterior pituitary gland under control of the nearby hypothalamus.

The thyroid hormones are important regulators of metabolism. They increase the body's usage of carbohydrates and lipids to make energy and this maintains body temperature. Thyroid hormones are important promoters of protein syn-thesis which is why they are essential for normal growth in children.

Disorders of thyroid function

These can basically be divided into two groups, those that increase and those that inhibit thyroid hormone production.

Hyperthyroidism is a condition where the thyroid gland releases abnormally high quantities of thyroid hormones into the blood. There are various types, the most common being **Grave's disease**, an auto-immune condition, and also benign **adenomas**, non-cancerous growths within the thyroid. Both of these conditions can result in a visible enlargement of the thyroid gland called a **goitre**, and in some cases **exophthalmia** (protruding eyeballs). Patients with hyperthyroidism have elevated temperatures, nervousness and an increase in appetite, linked paradoxically with a reduction in body weight.

Severe hyperthyroidism is referred to as thyrotoxicosis, which can lead to a **thyrotoxic crisis** or 'thyroid storm'. Treatment here is of a specialist nature involving IV fluids and corticosteroids – as well as some of the antithyroid drugs.

Hypothyroidism is another auto-immune problem of the thyroid that causes a reduction in the release of thyroid hormones. In extreme cases this can cause a condition called **myxoedema**. Patients have a reduced metabolism, are lethargic and often speak very slowly. Hypothyroidism can also be caused by a diet severely deficient in iodine but this is rarely seen in the UK.

Drugs used to treat disorders of thyroid function

There are two drugs used in the treatment of long-term hyperthyroidism, *carbimazole* and *propylthiouracil*. These drugs inhibit the release of thyroid hormones and can return levels to near normal in around four to eight weeks. Their mechanism is not fully understood, but they are believed to inhibit an enzyme in the thyroid gland involved in the production of thyroid hormones.

Iodine/iodide, also known a *Lugol's solution*, is another drug available for the treatment of thyrotoxicosis. It is also used prior to elective surgery for partial **thyroidectomy** (removal of part of the thyroid gland). In the body, Iodine is converted to its ionic form iodide (I^-) and high levels of iodide appear to interfere with the regulatory mechanism of the thyroid gland, resulting in a reduction in the release of thyroid hormones.

Hypothyroidism is treated with synthetic thyroid hormone in the form of *levothyroxine sodium*. This is basically thyroxine (T_4) which simply increases serum thyroxine levels. There are currently no drugs available that stimulate the body to increase its own production of thyroid hormones. *Liothyronine sodium* is a close relative of *levothyroxine* but is reserved for emergency cases of severe hypothyroidism.

A QUICK RECAP on the thyroid gland, disorders and associated drugs

- Thyroid hormones T_3 and T_4 are important regulators of the body's metabolic rate.

- In Grave's disease, which is the most common form of hyperthyroidism, elevated thyroid hormone levels can result in goitre, exophthalmus, nervousness and weight loss.

- *Carbimazole* and *propylthiouracil* inhibit the release of thyroid hormones by the thyroid gland.

- In hypothyroidism, the metabolic rate is much reduced, resulting in lethargy. Treatment is by *levothyroxine sodium*, effectively thyroxine (T_4).

RUNNING WORDS

Here are some of the technical terms that were included in this chapter. Read through them one by one and tick them off when you are sure that you know what they mean.

Adenoma p. 251	Amine hormones p. 232	Apoptosis p. 247
Adipose p. 234		Biguanides p. 239
α (alpha) glucosidase p. 239	Anterior pituitary p. 241	Biphasic insulins p. 238
		Bone matrix p. 246

REFERENCES AND FURTHER RECOMMENDED READING

All recommended websites are open access (but free registration is sometimes required).

The Committee on Safety of Medicines (CSM) – http://www.mhra.gov.uk/

NHS Website – http://www.nhs.uk/Conditions/

Diabetes UK – http://www.diabetes.org.uk/

NICE Guidelines on Diabetes – http://www.nice.org.uk/Guidance/CG66/

National Osteoporosis Society – https://www.nos.org.uk/

Your turn to try

Now you have finished reading through this chapter try answering these questions to see how much you have learned.

The answers to these questions are at the end of the book on page 287.

1 How do peptide hormones communicate with cells?

2 Which class of hormones binds to intracellular receptors?

3 How does the liver store glucose?

4 What is the role of *glucagon* in glucose regulation?

5 What are the key differences between Type 1 and Type 2 diabetes?

6 Ketoacidosis is a problem when cells are starved of sugar and can occur in diabetics whose blood sugar levels are high. Explain this apparent anomaly.

7 Why can drugs such as *gliclazide*, *tolbutamide* and *metformin* not be used in Type 1 diabetes?

8 Which ovarian hormones are dominant in the follicular and luteal phases of the female reproductive cycle?

9 What are the typical postmenopausal symptoms?

10 What are the roles of osteoblasts and osteoclasts in osteoporosis?

11 How do the bisphosphonates attenuate osteoporosis?

12 How do combined oral contraceptives prevent conception?

13 Why are combined oral contraceptives not recommended immediately after childbirth?

14 What potential problems are there in prescribing antibacterial drugs to a woman taking combined oral contraceptives?

15 Name two observable symptoms that may occur in hyperthyroidism.

Answers to questions on page 229

1 The pancreas.
2 Reduces blood sugar levels.
3 Oestrogen and progesterone.
4 Increases metabolism.
5 Follicle-stimulating hormone.

Chapter 11

Drugs used in the treatment of mental health and neurological disorders

AIMS

By the time you have finished the chapter you should be able to understand:

1 The **physiology** – the neurophysiological basis of common mental health and neurological disorders affecting the brain.
2 The **pharmacology** – the action of the major drug groups used in the treatment of common mental health and neurological disorders affecting the brain.

CONTENTS

The chapter contains some brief case studies and ends with self-test questions to enable you to ensure that you have understood the neurophysiological nature of mental health problems and the pharmacology of drugs used to treat those disorders.

IN PRACTICE

Mental health problems are more common amongst the population than many would think. The UK Office for National Statistics in its 2000 survey estimated that around one in six people at any one time are suffering from mental health problems. These will vary from mild **anxiety** to serious problems such as **schizophrenia** and **bipolar disorders** (manic depression). Eating disorders and postnatal depression can also be included under the umbrella of mental health problems. Another closely related group of illnesses that have a physiological effect on the brain (and often a psychological effect) are the **dementias** such as **Parkinson's** and **Alzheimer's** disease which are becoming increasingly common with our ageing population. **Epilepsy** is another common disorder that affects the brain resulting in periodic seizures.

Regardless of your area of clinical practice, it is highly likely that some of your patients or their close relatives will have some form of mental health or neurological problem and may well be on medication for that problem. Although the treatment of people with mental health problems involves many different therapies such as counselling and psychotherapy, **psychoactive** drugs are used extensively. Drugs that are used to treat neurological disorders of the brain have many similarities with those used to treat mental health disorders (which is why they have been included in the same chapter). This is why it is important that all clinical practitioners have a working knowledge of the various groups of drugs used to treat people with mental health and neurological problems, and especially how those drugs can cause their many side-effects and interactions.

Introduction

Since before recorded history, humans have used psychoactive drugs to induce changes in their mental state. These drugs were mostly obtained from plants and fungi found growing in the locality and were often imbued with sacred powers and used in rituals and ceremonies. This ability of organic substances to bring about changes in our perception has continued through the ages to the present day. Some of these ancient drugs such as opium and cocaine are now classed as illegal narcotics and heavy penalties await those who deal in them. However, this is a fairly recent phenomenon and in the early part of the twentieth century, both opium and cocaine were sold over the counter in vast numbers of patent medicines. Cocaine was even part of the original formula of a popular American non-alcoholic carbonated drink that still bears the remnants of the drug's name (although cocaine as an ingredient was withdrawn long ago).

The therapeutic use of these drugs for mental health problems also stretches back into history. In eighteenth-century Britain, **laudanum**, a mixture of opium and alcohol, was recommended for melancholy and the Austrian psychoanalyst, Sigmund Freud, used cocaine for depression. One would hope that modern synthetic mental health drugs would be far removed from narcotic derivatives, but despite them being much more specific in their action, many such as barbiturates and amphetamines continue to be used illegally for recreational purposes.

Mental health problems range from mild depression to serious psychoses and there are a wide range of drugs available to help with these problems. As we will see in this chapter, our understanding of the psychophysiological action of most of these drugs is fairly limited because our understanding of the workings of the brain is equally limited. There are many factors that contribute to psychological health and, in these more enlightened times, no one would argue that pharmaceuticals are the best and only way to help people with mental health problems. However, the drugs we are about to discuss do have a role in therapy and many people depend on these therapeutic psychoactive drugs to help them to live a reasonably normal and productive life.

WHERE ARE WE STARTING FROM?

In this chapter we will examine the physiological basis of mental health disorders, neurological disorders affecting the brain, and their associated drugs. Most problems that affect the brain are poorly understood, as is the mechanism of the drugs used to treat them. However, let's start with the usual short quiz to find out how much you know before we begin:

1 Name the outer layer of the brain responsible for advanced thought processes.

_____

2 Do emotions such as fear originate in the inner or outer sections of the brain?

_____

3 What type of chemicals are noradrenaline and dopamine?

_____

4 5-Hydroxytryptamine is another name for . . .?

_____

5 What is the name of the structure that transmits signals between neurons?

_____

Answers are at the end of the chapter on page 279.

How did you do? Don't worry if you found these questions a bit tough. The brain is a particularly complex structure, perhaps **the** most complex structure, so the associated neurophysiology is equally complex. However, we need to understand the basics in order to have some inkling of how mental health and associated drugs work, and we will cover those basics in the forthcoming chapter.

11.1   The neurophysiological basis of mental health and neurological disorders

The origins and mechanisms of most mental health problems are poorly understood. Some neurological disorders such as Alzheimer's and Parkinson's disease do have an identifiable pathology involving the formation of abnormal proteins or the degeneration of neurons in specific areas of the brain. Most mental health disorders, however, have no apparent physiological manifestation and a tissue sample from the brain of a sufferer would in most cases be no different from the tissue sample of an individual without that problem. Sometimes there is the suggestion that a particular receptor is over-or under-expressed, or there may be some slight difference in the density of neural tissue in a particular region of the brain, but the relevance of these small differences is as yet poorly understood. Genetics, life experiences, relationships, even illegal drugs can all have an influence on our mental health but the precise nature and consequence of that influence will vary between individuals and it is almost impossible to predict how these factors may result in a mental problem.

ANOTHER WAY TO PICTURE THIS

The brain is like the central processing chip in your computer. Sometimes programs seem to crash for no apparent reason. Turn the computer off and frequently the problem will have righted itself when you turn it on again. The chip is in some ways like the brain – there may be no identifiable damage but sometimes the software malfunctions.

While the mechanisms behind most mental health disorders are as yet poorly characterised, we do know that chemical imbalance is a contributory factor in some disorders because most of the drugs used to treat mental illness alter the balance of chemicals in the brain. In some disorders, the influence of drugs may be to over-ride processes rather than to correct imbalances, but either way, changing the chemical balance of the brain is a therapeutic strategy that can sometimes produce beneficial results.

Many mental health drugs seem to exert their effects on the sections of the brain that control emotions and feelings. These are generally areas deep within the brain, centred around the **basal ganglia** (Figure 11.1). Changing the chemical balance within these areas can have a profound effect on an individual's sense of well-being.

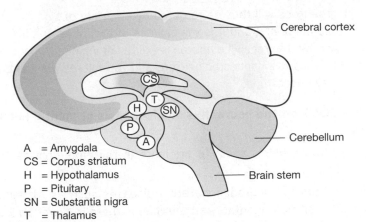

A = Amygdala
CS = Corpus striatum
H = Hypothalamus
P = Pituitary
SN = Substantia nigra
T = Thalamus

Figure 11.1 Section through the human brain showing some of the basal ganglia.

Basal ganglia are groups of nerve cells deep within the brain that control basic functions such as the autonomic nervous system, the endocrine system, movement, temperature control, etc.

When we discuss brain chemistry we are generally referring to the neurotransmitters released by synapses. We examined synapses in Chapter 6 where we saw how neurons communicate with each other by releasing neurotransmitters across a small gap between adjacent neurons called the synaptic cleft. These neurotransmitters can either stimulate or inhibit activity in their neighbouring cells. In the emotional centres deep within the brain, vast complex systems of neuronal relays interact with each other, sometimes stimulating and sometimes inhibiting, in a bewildering interplay of chemical activity. It is here that our mental health drugs produce their effect by changing the emphasis of stimulation or inhibition and somehow this tips the balance in the emotional brain, making the individual less anxious, less depressed, less prone to mood swings, etc. Precisely how this change in chemical activity translates into a change in mood or behaviour is at best poorly understood.

Neurotransmitters in the brain

There are many different types of neurotransmitter found in the brain. Some neurotransmitters such as **glutamate** and acetylcholine excite adjacent neurons whilst others such as **GABA**[1], **5-HT**[2] (**serotonin**) and **glycine** inhibit them. Noradrenaline and **dopamine** can be excitatory or inhibitory.

---

[1] GABA = gamma-aminobutyric acid.
[2] 5-HT = 5-hydroxytryptamine or serotonin.

The receiving neurons will thus be targeted by a variety of signals, some excitatory and some inhibitory, and it is the balance of excitation and inhibition that determines whether the receiving neuron is excited or inhibited. Imagine this happening in millions of interconnected neurons and you will see why the brain is still relatively poorly understood.

A QUICK RECAP on the neurophysiological basis of mental health disorders

- Mental health problems seem to originate in the emotional centres, deep within the brain.

- Except perhaps for neurodegenerative diseases such as Alzheimer's and Parkinson's, for most mental health problems there is as yet no identifiable physical pathology.

- Mental health problems are poorly understood but neurotransmitter imbalance may be a contributory factor because psychoactive drugs change the chemical balance in the synapses of the brain to produce their effect.

- Neurotransmitters can be either excitatory or inhibitory and it is the sum of excitatory and inhibitory signals on an individual neuron that determines whether it is excited or inhibited.

11.2 The principles of drug treatment for mental health and neurological disorders

Drugs used in mental health operate in or around the synapses deep within the brain. Before we examine their action in more detail, let us remind ourselves of the mechanisms taking place in the synapse. Figure 11.2 shows a typical synapse that might be excitatory or inhibitory – depending on the neurotransmitter that is being released. As a nervous impulse reaches the neuron terminal it causes the release of neurotransmitters from their prepacked vesicles. These neurotransmitters diffuse across the synaptic cleft and bind to receptors on the postsynaptic membrane of an adjacent neuron. When the receptors are activated they cause associated ion channels to open and (depending on the ion) the adjacent cell is either stimulated or inhibited. Whether the adjacent cell is stimulated enough to generate its own nervous impulse, depends on the sum of excitation and inhibition from all of the adjacent neurons.

Neurotransmitters quickly uncouple from their receptors and are either recycled back into the releasing neuron terminal through re-uptake transporters or de-activated by enzymes in the synapse. **Presynaptic receptors** on the neuron terminal respond to a variety of **neuromodulators**, chemicals that play a part in limiting the release of the neurotransmitters.

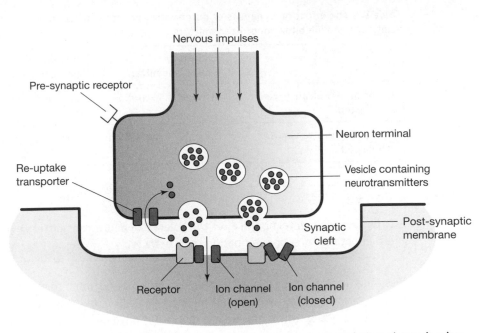

Figure 11.2 Synapse showing neurotransmitters binding to receptors and opening ion channels.

Drugs acting on the synapses of the brain do so in a variety of ways that we will discuss shortly but, essentially, by various means they lend either to **potentiate** or to **attenuate** the action of a particular neurotransmitter.

> To **potentiate** is to increase or amplify the activity of something and is the opposite of **attenuate**, which is to decrease its activity.

If the neurotransmitter is excitatory then potentiating its action shifts the synapse more towards excitation, whereas attenuating its action shifts the synapse away from excitation (towards inhibition). If the neurotransmitter is inhibitory then potentiating its action shifts the synapse more towards inhibition, whereas attenuating its action shifts the synapse away from inhibition (towards excitation). If that sounds rather complicated, Table 11.1 may explain it better.

ANOTHER WAY TO PICTURE THIS

Excitatory neurotransmitters are like the accelerator pedal on your car. If you potentiated the action of the accelerator, the car would go faster, but if you attenuated its action (perhaps cutting the accelerator cable), the car would slow down. Now compare the inhibitory neurotransmitters to your car's braking system. If you potentiated the action of the brakes, the car would slow down, but if you attenuated their action, the car would speed up.

Table 11.1 The effect on synapses of potentiating or attenuating the action of excitatory and inhibitory neurotransmitters

	Excitatory neurotransmitter	Inhibitory neurotransmitter
Action of neurotransmitter potentiated	Increase in excitation	Increase in inhibition
Action of neurotransmitter attenuated	Decrease in excitation	Decrease in inhibition

KEY FACT

Drugs used in mental health alter the balance of neurotransmitters in the brain, either potentiating or attenuating their activity.

Yes, this idea of drugs potentiating or attenuating inhibitory and excitatory neurotransmitters can appear rather puzzling at first, but it is an important principle in the action of mental health drugs. Sit down with a piece of scrap paper and work through it a few times – you will soon get the idea.

We will explain the action of the various drugs shortly but to demonstrate how central synapses are to their action, take a moment to examine Figure 11.3. This shows the site of action of the main groups of drugs used in mental health. You

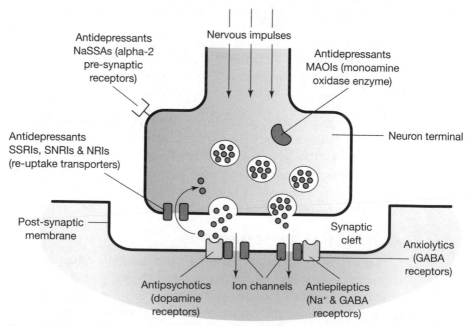

Figure 11.3 Structures in the synapses of the brain are the targets for the main drug groups used for mental health problems.

will see that all of the drugs interfere in some way with the workings of the synapse, either enhancing or inhibiting its action. It is important to note that the drugs highlighted in the figure will not all act on exactly the same synapse because many different classes of synapses are located in many different areas of the brain. However, it should help you to appreciate just how important a target the synapses are to mental health drugs.

We now arrive at the main problem in explaining the action of drugs used in the treatment of mental health disorders – namely, we do not fully understand how any of the drugs work! The reason for this is that we do not fully understand how the brain itself works. Neuroscientists have discovered much about the workings of the brain but there is much that remains a mystery. The brain is composed of billions of neurons interconnected by trillions of synapses that makes the most complex computer ever made look like a child's toy in comparison. We may know that a particular drug increases the concentration of a particular neurotransmitter in a particular area of the brain, but why it should relieve a feeling of depression is a matter of conjecture. Undoubtedly, techniques such as **PET** and **CAT** scans will enable us to explore more about the workings of the living brain. In the meantime, however, we have to admit that there is a large gap in our understanding between a drug's action in the synapse and its psychological effect on the patient.

> **KEY FACT**
> Our knowledge of the action of drugs used in mental health is by no means complete and we can only speculate how most may produce their psychological effect.

PET and **CAT scans** are nothing to do with vets, doggies and moggies but are acronyms for **Positron Emission Tomography** and **Computer Aided Tomography**. These non-invasive, high-tech imaging devices enable neurologists to examine the workings of the brain.

Mental health drugs and dependence

Most drugs that are used in mental health can cause dependence, similar in many aspects to the dependence some people develop on legal and non-legal drugs such as alcohol, nicotine and cocaine. The administration of a therapeutic drug may not produce a particularly pleasurable effect (as might illegal drugs) but withdrawal from it often causes discomfort or distress – especially if the individual has been taking the drug for a long time. The mechanisms that cause dependence are poorly understood. There may certainly be a biochemical basis for dependence, probably connected with the **limbic system**, an area of the brain concerned with emotions, mood and reward, but there is often a psychological element as well. Some drugs, especially the antipsychotic drugs, can produce acute withdrawal symptoms such as convulsions and confusion if the drug is discontinued suddenly. Hypnotics, anxiolytics and antidepressants can all cause dependence and are generally advised to be used for as short a period as possible to avoid this problem.

> The **limbic system** incorporates various basal ganglia and has a major but poorly understood role in the coordination of mood and emotions.

IN PRACTICE

Mental health drugs have the possibility of producing many side-effects and can cause dependence. As a general principle, mental health drugs should be prescribed cautiously, especially where an alternative, non-pharmacological treatment is available. If the drugs are prescribed, it should be for as short a period as possible.

A QUICK RECAP on the principles of drug treatment for mental health disorders

- Almost all drugs used for mental health disorders are targeted at synapses deep within the emotional centres of the brain.

- Drugs change the excitatory or inhibitory neurotransmitter balance in the synapses.

- Beyond their effect on the neurotransmitter balance in the synapses, we have relatively little understanding how most psychoactive drugs produce their psychological action.

- Many drugs used for mental health disorders can create dependence – both biochemical and psychological.

11.3 Drugs used in the treatment of mental health disorders

Mental health drug group 1: anxiolytics

Anxiety is not necessarily an abnormal state of mind and if you are in a stressful situation, such as a job interview, then it is perfectly normal to be anxious. These stressful situations result in a programmed series of physiological and psychological responses that include an increase in sympathetic activity, the release of stress hormones and an increase in alertness. This response is common to all mammals and prepares them for potential danger, and while a job interview is not particularly dangerous, it is still stressful and will provoke a stress response. Some people, however, suffer from anxiety brought about by situations that for most people would neither be stressful nor present a cause for concern or apprehension. This is unnatural anxiety that can often be helped by anxiolytics that relieve anxiety and help those with stress-related problems. They are not, however, appropriate for use in cases of depression, although some antidepressants such as *trazodone* are also licensed for anxiety.

The benzodiazepines are the main group of drugs used for the relief of short-term anxiety. They include *diazepam, alprazolam, chlordiazepoxide hydrochloride, lorazepam* and *oxazepam*. These drugs bind to a site on gamma-aminobutyric acid (GABA) receptors and enhance the inhibitory action of GABA. Because GABA receptors are widely distributed in the brain, the site of their action and the mechanism whereby they relieve anxiety is poorly understood. Beta-blockers such as *propranolol* are also licensed for use in anxiety but their action is predominantly physiological rather than psychological. However, reducing physical symptoms such as tremor and **palpitations** (disturbances in heart rhythm) can be reassuring for the patient and help to allay anxiety.

Side-effects for the anxiolytics are similar to those of the hypnotics (sleep inducers), drowsiness being the chief problem, which is why there is a caution for those driving or operating machinery.

> **DID YOU KNOW . . .** that beta-blockers such as *propranolol* and *atenolol* are banned in target sports such as archery and shooting as they steady the aim by reducing tremor and give the participants unfair advantage?

Mental health drug group 2: hypnotics

Hypnotics are prescribed for those suffering regularly from **insomnia** (lack of sleep). Drugs in this category include the benzodiazepines such as *nitrazepam, flurazepam, loprazolam, lormetazepam* and *temazepam. Zaleplon, zolpidem* and *zopiclone* are a closely related group of hypnotics that work in a similar manner to the benzodiazepines. If anxiety is a cause of the patient's insomnia then the anxiolytic benzodiazepine *diazepam* is sometimes used to treat both symptoms. The mechanism of action for the hypnotic benzodiazepines is the same as those used for anxiety alone.

Hypnotics are recommended for short-term use only for those with persistent insomnia.

As might be expected with drugs that send you off to sleep, drowsiness is one of the chief side-effects. Of course, this is a desirable action if the patient has retired to bed, but if the symptoms last over into the next day then this can present problems. *Nitrazepam* and *flurazepam* tend to have a longer duration of

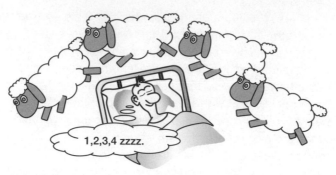

Figure 11.4 Non-pharmacological methods, e.g. relaxation techniques, etc., are preferred for those with persistent insomnia.

action compared to the other hypnotics mentioned above so would be avoided in patients who may be driving or operating machinery the following morning.

CASE STUDY

Zaheer is a successful businessman but recently he has been involved in stressful negotiations for an important contract. He is also worried about his son who is ill. He presents at your clinic with anxiety that he says is keeping him awake at night. What would you suggest?

Comment on case study Being anxious when your children are ill is perfectly normal and quite likely to cause insomnia, and Zaheer's sleep problems are likely to be compounded by his stressful work life. Before hypnotics or anxiolytics are prescribed, you might try to find out more about his home circumstances and the nature of his son's illness. Some men can find it quite difficult to discuss their problems but talking in confidence to a practitioner may help to allay Zaheer's anxieties. Find out what his evening routine is, does he allow himself time to unwind after work? If his problems appear to be short term then a hypnotic for a week or two might help him to get a good night's sleep, but preferably choose one that has a shorter duration of action so as not to interfere with his daytime activities. His anxiety is not a clinical problem because it is a normal response to a stressful situation, so you would be reluctant to prescribe an anxiolytic drug at this stage.

Mental health drug group 3: antidepressants

Depression is relatively common in our society and around 15 per cent of us will suffer from this problem at some time. Depression is more than being sad such as when a loved one dies: it is a clinical syndrome that can produce feelings of apathy, bleakness and lack of self-esteem – even when the individual may, to all intents and purposes, have acceptable domestic, social and financial circumstances. Psychological symptoms can also be accompanied by physical symptoms such as loss of appetite, tiredness and digestive problems. Postnatal depression is quite common in mothers of newly-born children.

As with all mental health problems, the pathophysiology of depression is poorly understood. We do know, however, that pharmacological interference in brain chemistry can, in many cases, improve the symptoms and often allows people afflicted with depression to live a relatively normal life. There are three main groups of antidepressants – **tricyclic antidepressants** (TCAs), **selective serotonin re-uptake inhibitors** (SSRIs) and **monoamine oxidase inhibitors** (MAOIs). There are also antidepressants – some of them recently introduced – that do not fit into a neat group so, in line with the *British National Formulary*, we will refer to them as 'other antidepressant drugs'.

Activity of the first three groups centres on serotonin (5-HT) and noradrenaline-releasing neurons in the brain. Both of these neurotransmitters are of the same monoamine chemical group and share the same re-uptake transporter. They are released from their neuron terminals and bind to receptors on the postsynaptic membrane where they have an inhibitory effect on that cell. The neurotransmitter then decouples from the receptor and is taken back via a re-uptake transporter protein in the presynaptic terminal. Here some of the neurotransmitters are degraded by the enzyme **monoamine oxidase** as part of the terminal's regulatory mechanism (Figure 11.5).

Tricyclic antidepressants (TCAs), such as *amitriptyline, imipramine* and *lofepramine*, are non-selective monoamine re-uptake inhibitors. They block the re-uptake transporters for 5-HT (serotonin) and noradrenaline so the neurotransmitters remain in the synaptic cleft, in other words, their concentration there is effectively increased. This means that there are more neurotransmitter molecules to bind to the receptors so the effect of the neurotransmitter is enhanced.

Selective serotonin re-uptake inhibitors (SSRIs), such as *fluoxetine, citalopram, escitalopram, fluvoxamine, paroxetine* and *sertraline*, are more specific for the re-uptake transporters of 5-HT and tend to exert their effects predominantly in 5-HT synapses.

Monoamine oxidase inhibitors, such as *phenelzine, isocarboxazid* and *tranylcypromine*, irreversibly inhibit the intracellular enzyme monoamine oxidase. This

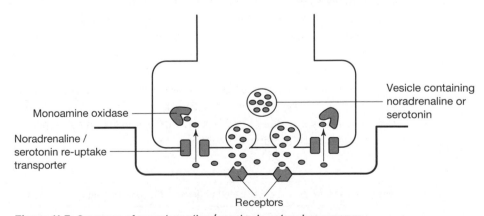

Figure 11.5 Synapse of noradrenaline/serotonin releasing neurons.

enzyme breaks down monoamines such as noradrenaline, dopamine and 5-HT. Inhibition of the enzyme therefore increases the concentration of these neuro-transmitters in the synapse. These drugs are less frequently used these days because of their potential side-effects and interactions (see below). Another member of the group, *moclobemide*, is a reversible inhibitor of the MAO enzyme and is claimed to have fewer side-effects.

Other antidepressant drugs

There are some drugs that do not easily fit into the main classes of antidepres-sants. Included in this 'group' are *duloxetine, flupentixol, mirtazapine, reboxe-tine, tryptophan* and *venlafaxine*.

- *Duloxetine* and *venlafaxine* – are used in the treatment of major depression. Both inhibit the re-uptake of serotonin and noradrenaline and are therefore referred to as **serotonin and noradrenaline re-uptake inhibitors** (SNRIs).

- *Reboxetine* – is used in the treatment of major depression. It is a selective inhibitor of the re-uptake of noradrenaline and is therefore referred to as a **noradrenaline re-uptake inhibitor** (NRI).

- *Flupentixol* – is a dopamine receptor antagonist that can also be used as an antipsychotic drug. It blockades dopamine receptors in the midbrain but can also affect motor neuron relays in the substantia nigra, which may explain the Parkinson-like problems of muscle control experienced by some patients.

- *Mirtazapine* – is used in the treatment of major depression. It is an **alpha-2 adrenergic receptor antagonist**, classified pharmacologically as a **noradren-ergic and selective serotonin antidepressant (NaSSA)**. These drugs are believed to work by blocking presynaptic alpha-2 adrenergic receptors that normally inhibit the release of noradrenaline and serotonin. This increases the avail-ability of these two neurotransmitters in the synapse and so has an effect similar to that of the SNRIs, *duloxetine* and *venlafaxine*.

- *Tryptophan* – is an amino acid that is converted via **5-hydroxytryptophan** into **5-hydroxytryptamine** (serotonin) – Figure 11.6. Administered as an anti-depressant drug, *tryptophan* works by increasing the production of serotonin. *Tryptophan* has been linked to **eosinophilia–myalgia syndrome**, a debilitating muscle problem caused by abnormally high levels of circulating white blood cells called eosinophils. However, there remains some debate as to whether this problem was actually caused by the drug or by impurities in the manufac-turing process. *Tryptophan* is not the drug of first choice for depression, but can be used as an adjunct under specialist supervision for depression that has resisted standard antidepressants.

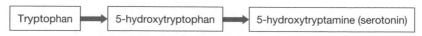

Figure 11.6 The synthesis of 5-hydroxytryptamine from tryptophan.

SSRI? SNRI? Yes indeed, all these acronyms can get somewhat confusing so let's list them again . . .

- **SSRI** – Selective Serotonin Re-uptake Inhibitor
- **SNRI** – Serotonin / Noradrenaline Re-uptake Inhibitor
- **NRI** – Noradrenaline Re-uptake Inhibitor
- **NaSSA** – Noradrenergic and Selective Serotonin Antidepressant

St John's Wort (*Hypericum perforatum*)

Up to this point we have resisted the inclusion of any unlicensed drug that does not appear in the *British National Formulary*. We are making an exception for St John's wort, firstly because there is good evidence that it relieves mild to moderate depression and secondly, although unlicensed, it does get a mention in the BNF (albeit for its interactions). A third reason for its inclusion here is because it is very popular with the public who see it as a safe, natural alternative to conventional antidepressant drugs. *Hypericum perforatum* is a small, rather scruffy, yellow-flowered plant that is common on uncultivated open ground. It gets its species name from the leaves that can be seen to have small perforations when held against the light. The leaves and flowers contain a myriad of organic chemicals including **hypericin, hyperforin**, various **flavonoids, tannins** and essential oils. It appears to exert its antidepressant effect mainly by inhibiting serotonin re-uptake transporters, in a similar way to *fluoxetine* and *paroxetine*. However, side effects from this herb are claimed to be fewer than with conventional SSRIs – although whether side-effects are dose-related is difficult to determine as the chemical composition of the raw herb can vary considerably between batches.

> **Flavonoids** are plant chemicals that have antioxidant properties and so are believed to be beneficial to human health, helping to prevent cancer and cardiovascular disease. **Tannins** give tea and wine their astringent flavour.

Side-effects of antidepressants

Each patient may react differently with regard to side-effects. The tricyclic antidepressants generally have a greater potential for side-effects than do the SSRIs because the TCAs are less selective and bind to both noradrenaline and 5-HT re-uptake transporters. Potential side-effects with these drugs include dry mouth, sedation, blurred vision, constipation, nausea, etc. TCAs also have the potential to cause arrhythmias, tachycardia and postural hypotension and their use is contra-indicated in patients with arrhythmias and those who have suffered a recent heart attack. SSRIs are less sedating and less likely to cause cardiovascular problems, their main side-effects being on the gastro-intestinal system where they can cause diarrhoea, nausea, dyspepsia, etc.

Like all substances that have a genuine pharmacological effect, *Hypericum perforatum* has side-effects and interactions. This herb can induce P450 enzymes

269

in the liver and increases the metabolism (and so reduces the plasma concentration) of various drugs, for example, anti-epileptics such as *carbamazepine*, cardiac glycosides such as *digoxin*, anticoagulants such as *warfarin*, oral contraceptives (both oestrogens and progestogens) and many more – see the BNF for a full list.

Monoamine oxidase inhibitors have their own range of unwanted effects such as dizziness and postural hypotension (especially in the elderly). A significant problem with MAOIs is that they interact with many other drugs and also some foods. The monoamine oxidase enzyme is distributed widely in the body where it breaks down a wide variety of nitrogenous molecules, including those ingested with food. Inhibiting monoamine oxidase with a MAOI drug can result in a build-up of **tyramine**, an amine that is found in foods such as mature cheese, soy sauce, game meats such as pheasants, as well as those perennial and uniquely British favourites, Bovril®, Oxo® and Marmite®. Tyramine can cause the release of noradrenaline from storage vesicles in sympathetic neurons resulting in vasoconstriction and tachycardia, which together can cause a dramatic increase in blood pressure, the so-called '**tyramine pressor response**'.

Drugs such as *Flupentixol* that blockade dopamine receptors have their own set of problems, associated with motor neuron relays in the basal ganglia that can result in problems with motor coordination.

Mental health drug group 4: antipsychotics

Antipsychotic drugs have a tranquilising and sedative effect on the mind and are used selectively for serious problems such as schizophrenia, severe anxiety and violent or unpredictably impulsive behaviour. Their use requires specialist knowledge in the field of mental health prescribing, so we will discuss them only briefly here. They can be divided into two groups, the **typical** and the newer **atypical** antipsychotics.

Most of the typical antipsychotics are of the **phenothiazine** group and include *chlorpromazine, levomepromazine, flupentixol, haloperidol, promazine* and *zuclopenthixol*. All of these drugs are dopamine antagonists that block D_2 dopamine receptors in the CNS, but precisely how this produces the effect of stabilising mood and feelings is poorly understood. Atypical anti-psychotics form a sub-group that includes *amisulpride, aripiprazole, clozapine, olanzapine, quetiapine, risperidone* and *zotepine*. These include some of the more recently introduced antipsychotics that are considered to be better tolerated than the older drugs. As with the typical antipsychotics, these drugs act by binding to synaptic dopamine receptors but may have less affinity for the motor neuron relays in the **substantia nigra**, which explains why some produce fewer side-effects related to motor coordination. Some in the group also appear to have an affinity for 5-HT (serotonin) receptors as well as alpha-2 adrenergic receptors, perhaps explaining other effects on mood.

Although most of these drugs are available in tablet form, in slow-release formulations, some can be given by **depot injections**. Drugs such as *flupentixol* *decanoate, fluphenazine decanoate, haloperidol* (as decanoate), *pipotiazine palmitate, risperidone* and *zuclopenthixol decanoate* may be administered every two to four weeks, which may help with patients whose compliance with oral medication is poor.

> **Depot injections** are given to patients for whom compliance may be a problem. The special formulations allow the drug to be released slowly from its site of injection (usually the buttocks) over a period of several weeks.

Side-effects of antipsychotics

Any drug that interferes with the normal working of the brain can be expected to have profound side-effects and the antipsychotics are no exception. Dopamine is an important neurotransmitter in areas of the brain, such as the substantia nigra, that are involved in control of movement and muscles. Blocking the action of dopaminergic relays with antipsychotic drugs can cause problems such as involuntary movements and symptoms similar to those in **Parkinson's** disease. Here, the degeneration of dopaminergic neurons in the substantia nigra produces **dyskinesia**, lack of motor coordination, difficulty walking, tremor, loss of facial expression, etc. Another cause of the many side-effects produced by this group of drugs is their tendency to bind to 5-HT, acetylcholine and noradrenaline receptors, causing problems such as hypotension, dizziness, drowsiness, headache, confusion, etc.

Mental health drug group 5: antimanic drugs

Mania is a state of psychosis where an individual experiences an extreme state of excitement and elevation, sometimes with delusions and often with great physical energy. It is often a facet of **bipolar** disorder where the mood of the individual can swing from mania to depression, which is why it used to be termed **manic-depression**.

Lithium is the main drug that is used both in the prophylaxis and treatment of mania. It can also be used for the prophylaxis of bipolar disorder and recurrent depression. Its mechanism of action has yet to be elucidated. Lithium levels need to be carefully monitored to avoid toxicity that may cause convulsions and damage the kidneys.

A QUICK RECAP on drugs used in the treatment of mental health disorders

- Anxiolytics such as *diazepam* and *lorazepam* relieve anxiety by enhancing the action of GABA receptors.

- Hypnotics induce sleep and include benzodiazepines such as *nitrazepam* and *temazepam*. Closely related to the anxiolytics, they have a similar mechanism of action.

- Antidepressants are divided into three main groups – tricyclic antidepressants (TCAs), selective serotonin re-uptake inhibitors (SSRIs) and monoamine oxidase inhibitors (MAOIs). They relieve depression by enhancing the action of 5-HT (serotonin) and noradrenaline.

- Other antidepressants include *duloxetine, flupentixol, mirtazapine, reboxetine, tryptophan* and *venlafaxine*. They have a variety of selectivity for 5-HT (serotonin), noradrenaline and dopamine activity.

- Antipsychotic drugs are divided into typical and atypical antipsychotics and have a tranquilising and sedative effect on the mind, mainly through the action of dopamine blockade. They tend to interfere with other receptors and have many side-effects.

- *Lithium* is the main drug used in both the prevention and treatment of mania.

11.4 Drugs used in the treatment of neurological disorders

So far we have examined disorders and drugs for mental health problems and we have broadly defined these as problems of the mind that affect people's mood and behaviour, but may not have an easily identifiable physiological origin. This section relates to physiological pathologies that affect the brain and often result in psychological disorders that may edge them towards the category of mental health problems. There are many different types of disorder that affect the brain, but we will concentrate on the three that are most common and have drugs associated with their treatment. Epilepsy results in periodic seizures while Parkinson's disease and Alzheimer's disease are termed dementias, a form of neurological deterioration that generally affects the elderly.

Drugs used in the control of epilepsy

Epilepsy is a neurological disorder – affecting over 450,000 people in the UK – that results in recurrent seizures (previously called fits). Some epilepsy has an identifiable origin such as a motor accident, a difficult birth or an infection such as meningitis, but for the majority of people the cause of their epilepsy is unknown. In reality, epilepsy is not one disease but various complex pathologies affecting different areas of the brain in different ways – but all resulting in some form of seizure. Some of theses seizures are apparently minor, resulting in confusion and an inability to speak while others can result in unconsciousness and convulsions. Sometimes the seizures arise for no apparent reason, but others have specific triggers such as flashing lights. Many people with epilepsy have few other symptoms beside their seizures and otherwise may live a normal life.

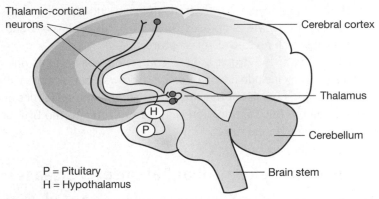

Figure 11.7 Uncontrolled discharges in the thalamic–cortical pathways are involved in epilepsy.

DID YOU KNOW . . . that some very famous people in history have suffered from epileptic seizures, including Julius Caesar, Napoleon Bonaparte, Leo Tolstoy, Lenin and Vincent van Gogh?

Epilepsy appears to be caused by uncontrolled discharges in the **thalamic–cortical** neurons that connect the thalamus and areas of the cerebral motor cortex (Figure 11.7). Generally the excitation of neurons is controlled by regulatory mechanisms in neural circuits that attenuate (damp down) neuronal activity and keep it confined to the immediate area. In epilepsy, however, this attenuation somehow malfunctions and neurons fire in a random and uncontrolled manner, affecting both the thalamus and cerebral cortex resulting in seizures, jerky muscle contractions and loss of consciousness.

All anti-epileptic drugs reduce excess neuronal activity in the brain, especially in the thalamic-cortical relays between the thalamus and the cerebral motor cortex. Drugs such as *carbamazepine* and *phenytoin* block Na^+ channels in high-frequency discharge neurons. *Ethosuximide* inhibits calcium ion channels in the relay of neurons between the thalamus and the cortex. Calcium ions entering neurons stimulate activity, therefore the blocking of Ca^{2+} channels damps down excessive neuronal activity in these areas.

Various anti-epileptic drugs centre their activity on GABA synapses in the thalamus. As GABA is an inhibitory neurotransmitter, enhancing its action will increase inhibition in the adjacent neurons which is beneficial when they are over-excited, as in epilepsy.

Valproate and *phenobarbital* (phenobarbitone) interact with GABA receptors, enhancing the opening of associated chloride channels which increases levels of inhibition in the thalamus. *Gabapentin*, despite its name, has relatively little affinity for GABA receptors and its mechanism is not fully understood. It is thought to act on presynaptic Ca^{2+} channels, possibly inhibiting the release of excitatory neurotransmitters such as glutamate and noradrenaline. *Vigabatrin* inhibits the

273

GABA-metabolising enzyme **GABA transaminase** and thus increases the availability of GABA. *Tiagabine* decreases GABA re-uptake into cells and thus more GABA is available to bind to GABA receptors.

The side-effects of the drugs used to control epilepsy are, as one might imagine, extensive. They include nausea, vomiting, drowsiness, dizziness, constipation, dry mouth, etc. For a full list of the side-effects of the anti-epileptics and all of the drugs mentioned in this section, you will need to refer to the BNF or data published by the drug manufacturer.

Drugs used in the control of Parkinson's disease

Parkinson's disease is a form of chronic neurological deterioration that affects around 120,000 people in the UK. It is generally a disease of old age that affects the substantia nigra, part of the basal ganglia that plays a role in coordinating movement. For reasons unknown, the dopamine-releasing neurons in this area start to die and this causes progressive deterioration, resulting in symptoms such as shaking, stiffness and slow movement. The problem also can result in loss of facial expression and everyday tasks such as speaking and writing may become difficult.

Because lack of dopamine is the major cause of problems in patients with Parkinson's disease, most treatments aim to increase dopamine levels in the brain.

Dopamine itself is unsuitable for use as a drug but its precursor *levodopa* is widely used in the treatment of Parkinson's disease. Unfortunately, before it reaches the central nervous system *levodopa* is quickly converted into dopamine by the enzyme **dopa-decarboxylase** and this results in dopamine-associated side-effects, including nausea and cardiovascular problems (Figure 11.8a). In order to overcome this problem, dopa-decarboxylase inhibiting drugs such as *benserazide* or *carbidopa* are combined with *levodopa* and this allows *levodopa* to enter the central nervous system where it is finally converted into dopamine and can exert its therapeutic effect (Figure 11.8b). *Benserazide* or *carbidopa* themselves are unable to cross the blood–brain barrier and so have no effect on the conversion of *levodopa* into dopamine in the central nervous system.

Dopamine receptor agonists include drugs such as *apomorphine, bromocriptine, cabergoline, pergolide, pramipexole, ropinirole* and *rotigotine*. These drugs mimic the action of dopamine in the motor relays of the central nervous system and restore some of the function caused by loss of dopaminergic neurons. These

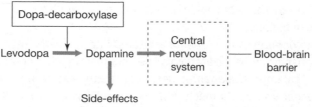

Figure 11.8a Outside the CNS *levodopa* is converted into dopamine by the enzyme dopa-decarboxylase.

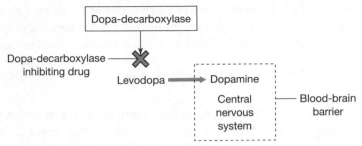

Figure 11.8b Dopa-decarboxylase-inhibiting drugs such as **benserazide** or **carbidopa** allow **levodopa** to enter the CNS where it is converted to dopamine.

drugs have fewer long-term complications with regard to motor coordination compared to **levodopa** but may produce more psychological side-effects such as confusion and hallucinations – especially those **ergot-derived** drugs such as **bromocriptine**, **cabergoline** and **pergolide**.

> **Ergot-derived** drugs are extracted from the *Claviceps* fungus that infects cereals and contains the alkaloid ergotamine that is used to synthesise the hallucinogenic drug LSD (which may possibly explain some of the side-effects).

Drugs used in the control of Alzheimer's disease

Alzheimer's disease is the most common form of dementia, affecting around 450,000 people in the UK, most of them over the age of 65. It is a progressive condition that starts with forgetfulness and difficulty remembering the right words. As the disease progresses the individual is subject to mood swings and confusion and eventually major changes in personality and behaviour can occur. The pathology of Alzheimer's disease is not well understood but it is known that there is a gradual loss of neurons and synapses, especially in the cerebral cortex. This is compounded by a build-up of abnormal proteins around the neurons and fibril tangles within the neurons. The production of the neurotransmitter acetylcholine is also affected.

There is no cure for Alzheimer's disease but drugs such as **donepezil**, **galantamine**, **memantine** and **rivastigmine** can slow the development of symptoms. **Donepezil**, **galantamine** and **rivastigmine** are inhibitors of the enzyme **acetylcholinesterase** that breaks down synaptic acetylcholine. Inhibiting this enzyme therefore reduces the rate of degradation of acetylcholine and thus synaptic levels of this neurotransmitter increase, partially compensating for a reduction in cholinergic activity. **Memantine** is an antagonist of the **NMDA (N-methyl d-aspartate)** glutamate receptors. Excessive amounts of this excitatory neurotransmitter are believed to overstimulate neurons, causing damage through a process called excitotoxicity that can result in cell death. By shielding the NMDA receptor from the effects of glutamate, *memantine* reduces excitoxicity, along with cell death. These drugs may delay the progression or alleviate the symptoms of Alzheimer's disease but it inevitably results in steady neurological deterioration and death.

A QUICK RECAP on drugs used in the treatment of neurological disorders

- Drugs used in the treatment of epilepsy have a variety of actions, most of which delay neural transmission in the thalamic–cortical pathways. *Carbamazepine* and *phenytoin* block Na^+ channels in high-frequency discharge neurons. *Valproate, vigabatrin, phenobarbital* and *tiagabine* increase the inhibitory effects of GABA.

- Parkinson's disease is primarily caused by a reduction in dopamine-releasing neurons in the basal ganglia of the brain that play an important part in motor coordination.

- Drugs used to treat Parkinson's disease such as *apomorphine, bromocriptine*, etc., are dopamine agonists that increase dopamine activity in the basal ganglia and restore some motor coordination. *Levodopa* is a precursor of dopamine that is converted to dopamine in the brain.

- Alzheimer's disease is an irreversible form of dementia whose pathology is not fully understood. Drugs such as *donepezil, galantamine* and *rivastigmine* increase the activity of acetylcholine activity in the brain and help with symptoms. *Memantine* reduces damage from excitotoxicity and helps to prevent the loss of neurons.

RUNNING WORDS

Here are some of the technical terms that were included in this chapter. Read through them one by one and tick them off when you are sure that you understand them.

Acetylcholinesterase p. 275

Alpha-2 adrenergic receptor antagonists p. 268

Alzheimer's disease p. 256

Anxiety p. 256

Attenuate p. 261

Atypical antipsychotics p. 270

Basal ganglia p. 258

Bipolar p. 271

Bipolar disorders p. 256

CAT scans p. 263

Dementia p. 256

Depot injections p. 270

Dopamine p. 259

Dopa-decarboxylase p. 274

Dyskinesia p. 271

Eosinophilia-myalgia syndrome p. 268

Epilepsy p. 256

Ergot-derived drugs p. 275

Flavonoids p. 269

GABA p. 259

GABA transaminase p. 274

Glutamate p. 259

Glycine p. 259

5-HT p. 259

5-Hydroxytryptamine p. 268

5-Hydroxytryptophan p. 268

Hyperforin p. 269

Hypericin p. 269

Insomnia p. 265

Laudanum p. 257

Limbic system p. 263

Manic – depression p. 271

Monoamine oxidase p. 267

Monoamine oxidase inhibitors (MAOIs) p. 267

Neuromodulators p. 260

NMDA – N-methyl d-aspartate p. 275

Noradrenaline re-uptake inhibitor (NRI) p. 268

Noradrenergic and selective serotonin antidepressant (NaSSA) p. 268

Palpitations p. 265

Parkinson's p. 256

PET scans p. 263

Phenothiazine p. 270

Potentiate p. 261

Presynaptic receptors p. 260

Psychoactive p. 256

Schizophrenia p. 256

Selective serotonin re-uptake inhibitors (SSRIs) p. 267

Serotonin p. 259

Serotonin and noradrenaline re-uptake inhibitors (SNRIs) p. 268

Substantia nigra p. 270

Tannins p. 269

Thalamic–cortical p. 277

Tricyclic antidepressants (TCAs) p. 267

Typical antipsychotics p. 270

Tyramine p. 270

Tyramine pressor response p. 270

REFERENCES AND FURTHER RECOMMENDED READING

All recommended websites are open access (but free registration is sometimes required).

Linde, K., Mulrow, C.D., Berner, M. and Egger, M. (2005) *St John's Wort for Depression*. The Cochrane Collaboration.

Office for National Statistics (2000) *Psychiatric Morbidity Among Adults Living in Private Households in Great Britain*.

MIND (mental health charity) – http://www.mind.org.uk/

Mental Health Foundation – http://www.mentalhealth.org.uk/

NHS website – http://www.nhs.uk/Conditions/

National Society for Epilepsy – http://www.epilepsynse.org.uk/

The Parkinson's Disease Society – http://www.parkinsons.org.uk/

The Alzheimer's Society – http://www.alzheimers.org.uk/

Your turn to try

Now you have finished reading through this chapter try answering these questions to see how much you have learned.

The answers to these questions are at the end of the book on page 287.

1 What is the name of the clusters of nerve cells deep within the brain that form the target for most mental health drugs?

2 GABA is short for . . .?

3 Are GABA, 5-HT and glycine inhibitory or excitatory neurotransmitters?

4 What is a re-uptake transporter and where is it situated?

5 What is the effect of potentiating the effect of an inhibitory neurotransmitter?

6 What is the effect of attenuating the effect of an excitatory neurotransmitter?

7 Which receptors are the main targets for anxiolytics such as the benzodiazepines?

8 What is the main side-effect of hypnotic drugs?

9 What is the main side-effect of drugs that block dopamine receptors?

10 Tricyclic antidepressants increase the concentration of which two neurotransmitters in the synaptic cleft?

11 Which group of drugs might be incompatible with Marmite® on toast?

12 What is the main concern taking *Hypericum perforatum* with conventional drugs?

13 What are the main group of receptors for antipsychotics?

14 Lithium is prescribed for which disorder?

15 Which neural pathways are targeted by anti-epileptic drugs?

Answers to questions on page 257

1 The cerebral cortex.
2 The inner section of the brain.
3 Neurotransmitters (catecholamines to be exact).
4 Serotonin.
5 The synapse.

General resources: books and websites

Useful reference books

Some of these books focus primarily on the use and administration of drugs in clinical practice rather than on pharmacological mechanisms, but as they all add to the reader's understanding of the subject they are worthy of mention.

Adams, M.P. *et al.* (2007) *Pharmacology for Nurses – A Pathophysiologic Approach* (2nd edition). Prentice Hall.

Coleman, M. (2006) *Drug Metabolism*. Wiley–Blackwell.

Galbraith, A. *et al.* (2007) *Fundamentals of Pharmacology* (2nd edition). Pearson Education.

Golan, D.E. *et al.* (2007) *Principles of Pharmacology* (2nd edition). Lippincott, Williams & Wilkins.

Greenstein, B. and Gould, D. (2009) *Trounce's Clinical Pharmacology* (18th edition). Churchill Livingstone.

McGavock, H. (2005) *How Drugs Work* (2nd edition). Radcliffe Publishing Ltd.

Rang, H.P. *et al.* (2007) *Rang and Dale's Pharmacology* (6th edition). Churchill Livingstone.

Useful websites

There is plenty of information on the Web but not all of it is reliable. Here are a few useful websites run by more reputable organisations – and with free access.

NHS Direct: Health encyclopaedia – This site contains some useful information on the symptoms, causes, diagnosis and treatment of a wide range of diseases – http://www.nhsdirect.nhs.uk/

Bandolier – UK website assessing the evidence base for the use of drugs and other treatments. Hosted by Oxford University – http://www.medicine.ox.ac.uk/bandolier/

The Cochrane Collaboration – Independent, non-profit-making organisation that evaluates clinical trials and publishes systematic reviews on drugs and other treatments – http://www.cochrane.org/

Student BMJ – Website maintained by the British Medical Journal. Primarily aimed at medical students, it contains useful articles on various aspects of medicine including diagnosis and treatment – http://student.bmj.com/

eMedicine is an open-access US-based website that provides extensive information on the nature and treatment of a wide range of diseases. Written by health professionals, the information is evidence-based, but note that information may not be in concordance with UK clinical protocols – http://emedicine.medscape.com/

RxList is an open-access US-based website that provides extensive information on therapeutic drugs. Information on generic drugs will be useful to UK practitioners but note that US dosages, prescribing protocols and the formulations of proprietary drugs may be different from those in the UK - http://www.rxlist.com/

Merck manuals - online medical library are maintained by the US pharmaceutical company, Merck & Co. Inc. This is an extensive database that provides detailed information on a wide range of conditions and their treatment. Note that information may not be in concordance with UK clinical protocols - http://www.merck.com/mmpe/index.html

Answers to 'Your turn to try'

Chapter 1, page 20

1 (a) Nucleus – contains the DNA that codes for proteins.
   (b) Ribosomes – assemble amino acids into proteins.
   (c) Mitochondria – produce ATP.
   (d) Cell membrane – controls the passage of materials in and out of the cell.
2 Lipid.
3 Receptors, ion channels, enzymes and carrier proteins.
4 A gene.
5 Amino acids.
6 An oil is liquid at room temperature whereas a fat is solid.
7 Cholesterol.
8 Starch
9 Fuel (glucose or lipids) and oxygen.
10 It is transported in the blood from the cells to the lungs where it is breathed out.

Chapter 2, page 42

1 20,000.
2 (1) There are many different types of protein.
   (2) Proteins have important roles in physiological processes.
   (3) Each organ and tissue has protein distinctive to that organ and tissue.
3 Hormones, neurotransmitters and mediators.
4 They are the appropriate shape for that receptor (right key for lock).
5 It is a similar shape/molecular structure to adrenaline.
6 An agonist drug binds to a receptor and has the same effect as the natural chemical messenger binding to that receptor. An antagonist drug binds to and blocks a receptor from its natural chemical messenger.
7 A sympathomimetic drug has an adrenergic effect, i.e. the same effect as stimulation by the sympathetic nervous system.
8 Acetylcholine.
9 Cations are *positively* charged ions.
10 Voltage-controlled ion channel
11 Stops the transmission of nervous impulses (action potentials) along the pain neurons.
12 The enzyme's active site.
13 The cholesterol synthesis pathway (in the liver)
14 A carrier protein requires energy in the form of ATP to transport ions across membranes.

Chapter 3, page 69

1 Antihypertensives that result in hypotension, anticlotting drugs such as warfarin and heparin that can cause haemorrhage, laxatives that can cause diarrhoea, etc.
2 The therapeutic (or unwanted effects) caused by the drug are directly proportional to the dose administered.
3 Increases the heart rate.

4 *Salbutamol* targets β_2 receptors in the bronchioles but may also bind to β_1 receptors on the heart and produce the same effects as adrenaline – tachycardia.

5 Kininases degrade bradykinin but if their action is blocked the bradykinin levels build up and irritate the lining of the lungs.

6 Calcium channel blockers inhibit the contraction of smooth muscle, including that found in the walls of the digestive tract. A reduction in peristalsis can result in constipation.

7 Anticancer drugs inhibit cell division. White blood cells which are constantly being produced by cell division in the bone marrow will be affected.

8 Enteral, parenteral and topical.

9 Drugs pass from the gut into the hepatic portal vein and into the liver from where they are released into the circulatory system via the hepatic vein.

10 *Insulin* is a protein so is broken down by digestive enzymes (proteases).

11 GTN is almost completely metabolised during its initial passage through the liver and insufficient emerges into the blood to be of therapeutic value.

12 The initial metabolism of an orally ingested drug as it passes through the liver.

13 Most likely to increase in their bioavailability as P450 enzymes generally inactivate drugs so their inhibition will slow the rate of inactivation – and so increase bioavailability.

14 The level of drug in the blood that is greater than the minimum effective concentration but less than the maximum safe concentration.

15 The time it takes a drug to fall from 100 per cent of its concentration in the blood by one half, to 50 per cent concentration.

Chapter 4, page 108

1 Transport of nutrients, gasses, wastes, metabolites and hormones plus repair, thermoregulation and immunity.

2 Capillaries.

3 Coronary arteries.

4 Cholesterol.

5 Blood supply is reduced so insufficient oxygen is available to heart muscle cells. These cells start to produce lactic acid and this stimulates pain receptors.

6 More blood and oxygen is supplied to the heart muscle cells so they do not produce lactic acid.

7 A thrombus forming, possibly leading to a heart attack

8 A slower heart rate reduces the workload of the heart and so reduces angina pain.

9 Low-density lipoprotein (LDL).

10 The hepatocytes of the liver synthesise cholesterol to make good the shortfall.

11 HMG CoA reductase is an enzyme involved in the production of cholesterol in the liver. Inhibiting HMG CoA reduces cholesterol production, so the liver pulls in LDL cholesterol from the blood, thus lowering circulating levels of LDL.

12 Platelets, fibrin and red blood cells.

13 Aspirin inhibits the enzyme COX-1 in platelets and so reduces the production of thromboxane-A2, a mediator that increases the expression of GPIIb/IIIa receptors on platelets. These receptors bind with fibrin to form the mesh-like structure that makes up a blood clot.

14 Warfarin inhibits the process that produces the proteins involved in the clotting cascade. Heparins block the clotting cascade itself.

15 To break up a clot that has formed in the coronary arteries and is causing a heart attack.

Chapter 5, page 136

1 Yes, heart rate and pulse are the same.
2 Systole is the higher pressure.
3 Blood pressure falls.
4 Angiotensin-II, ADH-vasopressin and adrenaline.
5 Noradrenaline.
6 Heart rate would increase via the baroreceptor response.
7 BP falls because SVR has fallen.
8 Vasoconstriction, stimulation of ADH-vasopressin release, increase in blood sodium levels (and therefore blood volume and stroke volume).
9 With lower aldosterone levels, the kidneys retain less sodium so blood sodium levels fall. This reduces blood volume, stroke volume, cardiac output and so blood pressure.
10 Diuretics decrease the water reabsorbed so more urine is produced.
11 Hyponatraemia - more sodium is lost in the urine.
12 Contraction of the smooth muscle is reduced and this causes vasodilation of the arterioles.
13 CCBs also block calcium channels in the smooth muscle of the gut wall, inhibiting their contraction so causing a general reduction of gut motility.
14 Probably by reducing renin release so renin-angiotensin system inhibited.
15 Beta-blockers may block β_2 receptors in the lungs - the targets for bronchodilators such as salbutamol.

Chapter 6, page 161

1 'Pain is whatever the patient informs you that they are experiencing'.
2 Neuropathic.
3 Chronic.
4 Painful stimuli such as heat, mechanical pressure and chemical stimulation.
5 The painful stimulus detected by nociceptors and nervous impulses is sent along nociceptive neurons in the arm to the spinal cord. Impulses arrive via dorsal horn and synapse with ascending neurons that synapse with corticothalamic neurons in the thalamus. From here they travel to the cerebral cortex.
6 Opioid-like peptides are released during injury and block transmission between nociceptive neurons, so inhibiting the experience of pain.
7 Inflammation manifests itself by the following symptoms - redness, heat, swelling, pain and alteration of function
8 Histamine causes vasodilation and an increase in permeability of the small blood vessels.
9 Phospholipids - arachidonic acid - cyclic endoperoxides - prostaglandins and thromboxanes.
10 Cyclo-oxygenase 2.
11 PGE_2 causes vasodilation and (along with histamine) increases the permeability of small blood vessels, resulting in swelling and pain. PGE_2 also sensitises nociceptive neurons to the painful stimulation of bradykinin.
12 NSAIDs target COX-2 produced in inflammation but may also bind to and inhibit COX-1, an enzyme involved in the synthesis of non-inflammatory prostaglandins that maintain and protect the gastric mucosa (the lining of the stomach).
13 Because it can damage the liver.
14 Nausea, vomiting, respiratory depression, drowsiness and constipation.
15 Local anaesthetics block sodium ion channels in nociceptive neurons that are involved in the transmission of nervous impulses. If the nervous impulse is blocked from travelling to the brain, there will be no awareness of pain from the surgical procedure.

Chapter 7, page 180

1 Duodenum, jejunum and ileum.
2 Fatty acids.
3 Amylase.
4 Gastro-oesophageal and pyloric sphincters.
5 Pepsin.
6 Acetylcholine, histamine and gastrin.
7 Pancreas.
8 Gastro-oesophageal reflux disease (GORD).
9 *Helicobacter pylori*.
10 Constipation – increased passage time allows more time for reabsorption of water.
11 They form a raft that floats on top of the acidic stomach contents, protecting the oesophagus.
12 Histamine H_2 receptors.
13 PPIs block the pumping of H+ (protons) into the lumen of the stomach. There H+ normally combines with Cl– to form hydrochloric acid.
14 Opiates.
15 They pull water into the large intestine by osmosis, thus softening the stools and making their evacuation easier.

Chapter 8, page 205

1 Bacteria, viruses, fungi and protozoa.
2 Bacteria.
3 Bacteria are prokaryotes, meaning they do not have a true nucleus. All other organisms such as plants, animals and fungi are eukaryotic with true nuclei.
4 Cell wall, shape and oxygen requirement.
5 Peptidoglycan.
6 They inhibit the enzyme transpeptidase that produces peptidoglycan. This weakens the cell wall and the organism lyses.
7 They produce beta-lactamase enzymes that attack and denature the drugs.
8 It acts as a substrate for beta-lactamase, blocking its action so allowing the antibacterial drugs to kill the bacteria.
9 A bactericidal drug kills bacteria while a bacteriostatic drug prevents the bacteria from dividing.
10 Bacterial ribosomes.
11 They bind to calcium so may interfere with calcium supplies to the growing foetus.
12 Ergosterol, a sterol found in fungal cell membranes.
13 They have little in the way of structure to target and reproduce inside human cells which makes it difficult for drugs to reach them.
14 Vaccination.
15 *Metronidazole* is indicated for trichomoniasis and anaerobic bacterial infections.

Chapter 9, page 225

1 Mouth, trachea, bronchi, bronchioles, alveoli.
2 Around 80 m^2 or the area of half a tennis court.
3 The rate and depth of breathing increase.
4 In the medulla in the brain stem.
5 Long-term COPD patients switch from carbon dioxide to oxygen as the main driver of breathing.

6 Mucus traps bacteria and detritus and moves them out of the lungs.

7 Dust mites, pet hair, pollen, exercise, cold weather.

8 Shortness of breath.

9 In emphysema the walls of the alveoli break down, and in bronchitis excess mucus is trapped in the lungs leading to infections.

10 Smoking.

11 Smooth muscle cells surrounding the bronchioles.

12 Acetylcholine muscarinic receptors.

13 They suppress the activity of mast cells which release inflammatory mediators and eosinophils that damage the bronchial epithelium.

14 Corticosteroids inhibit protein synthesis and thus stunt growth.

15 Constipation.

Chapter 10, page 254

1 They bind to receptors on the cell surface.

2 Steroid hormones.

3 As glycogen, a polymer of glucose.

4 It stimulates the liver to break down glycogen into glucose which it releases into the bloodstream.

5 Type 1 diabetes is an autoimmune disease that destroys the beta islet cells of the pancreas so they cannot produce insulin. Type 2 diabetes usually occurs later in life and cells of the body become less sensitive to insulin, so their uptake of sugar falls. With time, insulin production may also be affected.

6 Diabetes is a disease caused either by lack of insulin or the cells' inability to take up glucose from the blood. This means that blood glucose levels can be abnormally high while intracellular glucose levels can be abnormally low. This can result in the cells switching to lipids for their fuel and producing acid ketones as a by-product.

7 These drugs rely on the beta cells of the pancreas having some residual insulin-producing capacity. In Type 1 diabetes these cells are destroyed, so cannot produce any insulin (which is why patients rely on insulin injections).

8 Oestrogen is the dominant ovarian hormone in the follicular phase and progesterone in the luteal phase.

9 Hot flushes, vaginal dryness, loss of sexual drive and mood swings.

10 Over-activity of the osteoclasts increases bone reabsorption and under-activity of the osteoblasts reduces bone reconstruction. This results in a net shift towards bone reabsorption so bones become weaker.

11 Bisphosphonates are incorporated into the bone matrix from where they are taken up by osteoclasts as they reabsorb bone. The bisphosphonates cause apoptosis (programmed cell death) in the osteoclasts so shifting the balance towards bone-building.

12 They mimic the hormonal environment of pregnancy which inhibits ovulation.

13 They interfere with lactation so are unsuitable if the woman is breast-feeding.

14 Some antibacterial drugs can interact with combined oral contraceptives, reducing their blood concentration and so reducing their effectiveness.

15 Goitre (swelling of the thyroid gland), exophthalmus (bulging eyeballs), nervousness and loss of weight.

Chapter 11, page 279

1 Basal ganglia.

2 Gamma-aminobutyric acid.

3 All inhibitory neurotransmitters.

4 Re-uptake transporters are situated in the presynaptic membrane. They are responsible for removing neurotransmitters from the synaptic cleft.

5 Greater inhibition.

6 Less excitation.

7 GABA receptors.

8 Drowsiness.

9 Problems with motor coordination, i.e. Parkinson-like symptoms.

10 5-HT and noradrenaline.

11 Monoamine oxidase inhibitors.

12 It can interact with conventional drugs such as warfarin to reduce their serum concentrations.

13 Dopamine (specifically D_2) receptors.

14 Mania and bipolar disorders.

15 Thalamic–cortical pathways.

Index

DATE DUE

Jan. 2/2012	
MAR 2 7 2015	